Nursing Skills and Practice:
A Process Approach

Nursing Skills and Practice: A Process Approach

Lacey Serrano

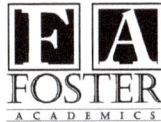

FOSTER
ACADEMICS

www.fosteracademics.com

www.fosteracademics.com

FA
FOSTER
ACADEMICS

Cataloging-in-Publication Data

Nursing skills and practice : a process approach / Lacey Serrano.
    p. cm.
Includes bibliographical references and index.
ISBN 978-1-63242-589-8
1. Nursing. 2. Practical nursing. 3. Medicine. I. Serrano, Lacey.
RT41 .N87 2019
610.73--dc23

Foster Academics,
118-35 Queens Blvd., Suite 400,
Forest Hills, NY 11375, USA

ISBN 978-1-63242-589-8 (Hardback)

Contents

Preface

Nursing is a profession in the domain of health care that deals with the provision of care and assistance to individuals, families or groups for the attainment of a good quality of life and optimal health. It involves the development of a plan of care for the treatment of illness, depending on an assessment and diagnosis of needs, outcomes and interventions and an evaluation of the outcomes of care. It can extend to assistance in activities of daily living, administering medicines and effective patient education. This book provides comprehensive insights into the vocation of nursing, its skills and practices. Such selected concepts that redefine this field have been presented herein. Coherent flow of topics, student-friendly language and extensive use of examples make this book an invaluable source of knowledge.

To facilitate a deeper understanding of the contents of this book a short introduction of every chapter is written below:

Chapter 1- The health care profession that focuses on the care of individuals, families or communities for the maintenance and recovery of health and quality of life is termed as nursing. This is an introductory chapter which will discuss briefly all the significant aspects of health care, nursing, nursing theory and nursing process.

Chapter 2- A nurse is an important health care professional who is entrusted with a number of responsibilities. These include bed management, bed-making, routine mouth care, morning care and respite care. These have been elaborately discussed in this chapter.

Chapter 3- The gathering of information pertaining to a patient's physiological, sociological, psychological and spiritual health by a registered nurse is referred to as general assessment. All the diverse aspects related to the types and techniques of nursing assessment have been carefully analyzed in this chapter.

Chapter 4- An examination and measurement of a patient's vital signs such as body temperature, pulse, blood pressure and respiratory rate is called a vital assessment. It is an important area of nursing assessment. This chapter discusses all aspects of vital assessment performed by a nurse through an analysis of the major vital signs and their assessment techniques.

Chapter 5- The medical investigation of a person's body in search of any signs or symptoms of a disease falls under physical examination. This chapter provides an overview of physical examination and the head-to-toe assessment of a patient that a nurse undertakes to gather crucial information regarding the patient's health.

Chapter 6- Activities of daily living(ADLs) refer to the daily self-care activities of a person. The assessment of ADLs in individuals post an injury or trauma, or suffering from a disability or age, allows information regarding their functional status. In order to completely understand activities of daily living, it is necessary to understand the processes related to it. The following chapter elucidates the varied processes and mechanisms associated with this area of study.

Chapter 7- The administration of medication to people suffering from a disease or diseases falls in the domain of medication administration. This chapter discusses in detail the diverse aspects and procedures involved in medication administration, such as rights and routes of medication administration.

Chapter 8- The interdisciplinary branch of medicine that uses different approaches to ease the suffering and improve a person's quality of life is known as pain management. This chapter explores the fundamentals and practices of interventional pain management, acupuncture, transcutaneous electrical nerve stimulation, etc.

Chapter 9- End-of-life care is the health care of a terminally ill person when the medical condition in its advanced stage, or of any individual in the final hours or days of his life. This chapter has been carefully written to provide an understanding of nursing care to a person near death. It includes the topics like palliative care, hospice care and spiritual care.

Chapter 10- Specimen collection, handling and preparation are important tasks performed by a nurse. Gathering samples in a way that ensures self-protection and prevents the spread of diseases is part of a nurse's core responsibilities. The topics elaborated in this chapter address the role of nurses in specimen collection, its techniques of handling, etc.

Chapter 11- The first stage in the treatment of any wound or a physical injury is in the evaluation of the cause, type and depth of the wound. The treatment involves cleaning, closing and dressing the wound. The management of wounds is an area of nursing care. This chapter explores the diverse aspects of wounds, wound care, wound first aid and wound care dressing.

Chapter 12- Assistive technology can help to improve the quality of life for patients with disabilities by allowing them greater independence for performing tasks that they cannot perform under normal circumstances. These technologies assist individuals with visual impairments, mobility impairments, eating impairments, etc. This chapter covers the use of patient assistive devices for walking, bathing, toileting, alternative communication devices, etc. and the role of nursing in assisting people who require such technologies.

Chapter 13- The nutrition of patients plays a crucial role in maintaining a healthy energy balance. It must be replete with the essential nutrients that speed up recovery. The routes of administration are oral, enteral or intravenous. This chapter studies the role of a nurse in patient nutrition and the basics of patient nutrition and hospital food.

Chapter 14- Perioperative care is the care provided to a patient before, during and after a patient's surgical procedure. Accordingly, it is divided into preoperative, peroperative and postoperative care. This chapter explores the essentials of perioperative care and the role of nurses during the perioperative period.

Chapter 15- The care of pregnant mothers prior to childbirth, during and after childbirth is essential to her health and safety as well as that of the newborn. Neonatal nursing or care for infants is a specialty of nursing care. Dealing with prematurity, infection, birth defects, surgical and cardiac malformations are also part of neonatal care. Nurses are vital to the deliverance of reproduction care and neonatal care. This chapter has been written to provide an extensive understanding of reproduction care and neonatal care and the role of nursing in providing it.

Chapter 16- Patient health records help to reduce errors related to prescription drugs, preventive and emergency care, and tests and procedures for ensuring patient safety. Keeping checks for drug-food interactions, allergies, drug dosages, patient information, etc. are all encompassed in patient health records. This chapter includes vital information on patient record maintenance for patient safety and discusses the aspects of medical error, electronic health record, evidence-based medicine, etc.

I would like to share the credit of this book with my editorial team who worked tirelessly on this book. I owe the completion of this book to the never-ending support of my family, who supported me throughout the project.

Lacey Serrano

Introduction to Nursing

The health care profession that focuses on the care of individuals, families or communities for the maintenance and recovery of health and quality of life is termed as nursing. This is an introductory chapter which will discuss briefly all the significant aspects of health care, nursing, nursing theory and nursing process.

Health Care

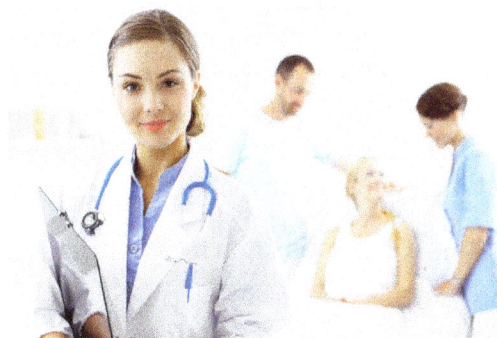

Healthcare is the act of taking preventative or necessary medical procedures to improve a person's well-being. This may be done with surgery, the administering of medicine, or other alterations in a person's lifestyle. These services are typically offered through a health care system made up of hospitals, physicians and nurses.

Types of Healthcare

Every individual has required different care depending upon their health problem like some require normal care and some require extra special care. So on the basis of patient condition healthcare divides into various types. The common types of healthcare are mentioned below.

Primary Healthcare

Primary health care mainly focuses on health equity producing social policy beyond the traditional healthcare system. Its main aim is to provide local care to a patient because professionals related to primary care are normal generalists, deals with a broad range of psychological, physical and social problems etc rather than specialists in any particular disease area. Primary care services rapidly increasing in both the developed and developing countries depending upon the increasing number of adults at greater risk of chronic noncommunicable disease like diabetes, asthma, back pain, hypertension, anxiety, depression etc.

To achieve the ultimate goals of primary health care., WHO has described five elements to achieve this goal. Following are:

- Stakeholder participation increased.

- Integrate health into all sectors.

- According to people need & expectation organizing healthy services.

- Pursuing collaborative models of policy dialogue.

Secondary Healthcare

This healthcare is provided by the medical specialists and other health problems who do not have direct contact with a patient like urologists, dermatologists, cardiologists etc. According to National health system policy, the patient required primary care professionals referral to proceed further for secondary care. Depends on countries to countries, the patient cannot directly take secondary care because sometimes health system imposed a restriction of referral on a patient in terms of payment.

The systems come under this category is known as District Health system and County Health system:

a. District Health system: This system mainly focus on child health and maternity care. People population of this system is about 25000 to 50000 and includes various healthcare centres and district hospitals. Healthcare centres receive referrals from various primary health care and is remain open for 24 hours every day. District hospitals include emergency services, neonatal care, comprehensive emergency obstetric etc and is remain open for 24 hours every day.

b. County Health system: Into this system, hospitals receive referrals from the District & community health systems. County hospital provides gynecologic services, general medicine, obstetrics, general surgery etc and is remain open for 24 hours every day.

Tertiary Healthcare

This type of healthcare is known as specialized consultative healthcare usually for in-patients and on referral from primary and secondary healthcare for advanced medical investigation and treatment. Examples of tertiary care services are plastic surgery, burn treatment, cardiac surgery, cancer management, neurosurgery, complex medical and surgical interventions etc.

The main provider of tertiary care is national health system consist of regional hospitals and national Hospital. Regional hospitals receive a reference from various county hospitals and serves as training sites complementary to the national referral hospital. It also provides additional care services and remains open for 24 hours every day.

Nursing

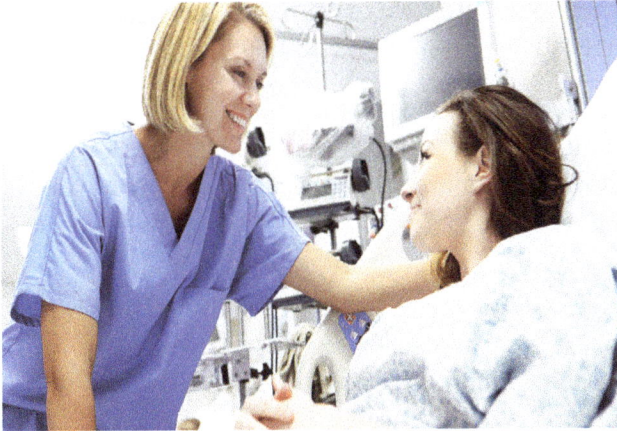

Nursing is a profession or practice of providing care for the sick and infirm. Nurses play an essential role in the healthcare industry, because they are primarily focused on patient care. They work in a variety of specialties to help people improve their health, and to prevent and heal illnesses and injuries.

Essential Characteristics of a Nurse

Communication Skills

Solid communication skills are a basic foundation for any career. But for nurses, it's one of the most important aspects of the job. A great nurse has excellent communication skills, especially when it comes to speaking and listening. Based on team and patient feedback, they are able to problem-solve and effectively communicate with patients and families.

Nurses always need to be on top of their game and make sure that their patients are clearly understood by everyone else. A truly stellar nurse is able to advocate for her patients and anticipate their needs.

Emotional Stability

Nursing is a stressful job where traumatic situations are common. The ability to accept suffering and death without letting it get personal is crucial. Some days can seem like non-stop gloom and doom.

That's not to say that there aren't heartwarming moments in nursing. Helping a patient recover, reuniting families, or bonding with fellow nurses are special benefits of the job. A great nurse is able to manage the stress of sad situations, but also draws strength from the wonderful outcomes that can and do happen.

Empathy

Great nurses have empathy for the pain and suffering of patients. They are able to feel compassion and provide comfort. But be prepared for the occasional bout of compassion fatigue; it happens to the greatest of nurses. Learn how to recognize the symptoms and deal with it efficiently.

Patients look to nurses as their advocates — the softer side of hospital bureaucracy. Being sympathetic to the patient's hospital experience can go a long way in terms of improving patient care. Sometimes, an empathetic nurse is all patients have to look forward to.

Flexibility

Being flexible and rolling with the punches is a staple of any career, but it's especially important for nurses. A great nurse is flexible with regards to working hours and responsibilities. Nurses, like doctors, are often required to work long periods of overtime, late or overnight shifts, and weekends.

Know that it comes with the territory. The upside is that a fluctuating schedule often means you're skipping the 9 to 5, cubicle treadmill. Sounds perfect, right? Run errands, go to the movies, or spend time with the family — all while the sun still shines.

Attention to Detail

Every step in the medical field is one that can have far-reaching consequences. A great nurse pays excellent attention to detail and is careful not to skip steps or make errors.

From reading a patient's chart correctly to remembering the nuances of a delicate case, there' s nothing that should be left to chance in nursing. When a simple mistake can spell tragedy for another's life, attention to detail can literally be the difference between life and death.

Interpersonal Skills

Nurses are the link between doctors and patients. A great nurse has excellent interpersonal skills and works well in a variety of situations with different people. They work well with other nurses, doctors, and other members of the staff.

Nurses are the glue that holds the hospital together. Patients see nurses as a friendly face and doctors depend on nurses to keep them on their toes. A great nurse balances the needs of patient and doctor as seamlessly as possible.

Physical Endurance

Frequent physical tasks, standing for long periods of time, lifting heavy objects (or people), and performing a number of taxing maneuvers on a daily basis are staples of nursing life. It's definitely not a desk job.

Always on the go, a great nurse maintains her energy throughout her shift, whether she's in a surgery or checking in on a patient. Staying strong, eating right, and having a healthy lifestyle outside of nursing is important too.

Problem Solving Skills

A great nurse can think quickly and address problems as — or before — they arise.

With sick patients, trauma cases, and emergencies, nurses always need to be on hand to solve a tricky situation. Whether it's handling the family, soothing a patient, dealing with a doctor, or managing the staff, having good problem solving skills is a top quality of a great nurse.

Quick Response

Nurses need to be ready to respond quickly to emergencies and other situations that arise. Quite often, health care work is simply the response to sudden incidences, and nurses must always be prepared for the unexpected.

Staying on their feet, keeping their head cool in a crisis, and a calm attitude are great qualities in a nurse.

10. Respect

Respect goes a long way. Great nurses respect people and rules. They remain impartial at all times and are mindful of confidentiality requirements and different cultures and traditions. Above all, they respect the wishes of the patient him- or herself.

Great nurses respect the hospital staff and each other, understanding that the patient comes first. And nurses who respect others are highly respected in return.

Barrier Nursing

The term "barrier nursing" is given to a method of nursing care that has been used for over one hundred years when caring for a patient known or thought to be suffering from a contagious disease such as open pulmonary tuberculosis. It is sometimes called "bedside isolation." As the name implies, the aim is to erect a barrier to the passage of infectious pathogenic organisms between the contagious patient and other patients and staff in the hospital, and thence to the outside world. Preferably, all contagious patients are isolated in separate rooms, but when such patients must be nursed in a ward with others, screens are placed around the bed or beds they occupy. The nurses wear gowns, masks, and sometimes rubber gloves, and they observe strict rules that minimize the risk of passing on infectious agents. All equipment and utensils used to care for the patient are immediately placed in a bowl of sterilizing solution, and attending nurses observe surgical standards of cleanliness in hand washing after they have been attending the patient. Bedding is carefully moved in order to minimize the transmission of airborne particles, such as dust or droplets that could carry contagious material, and is cleansed in special facilities that include the use of steam heat for sterilization.

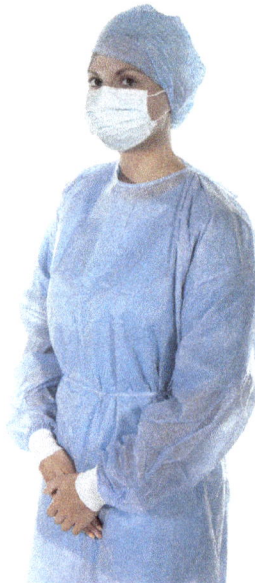

Barrier nursing often failed its objective, especially in hospital wards of the traditional "Nightingale" pattern, with rows of beds lined up on two or more sides of a large room. Airborne and droplet infection all too frequently penetrated the imperfect barrier, and sometimes even fecal-oral infectious agents found ways to invade the imperfect protective measures intended to block their passage. Late in the twentieth century, barrier nursing was superceded by more effective and more rigorous universal precautions.

Simple vs Strict Barrier Nursing

Simple Barrier Nursing

Simple barrier nursing is used when an infectious agent is suspected within a patient and standard precautions aren't working. Simple barrier nursing consists of utilizing sterile: gloves, masks, gowns, head-covers and eye protection. Nurses also wear Personalized protective equipment(PPE) to protect their bodies from infectious agents. Simple barrier nursing is often used for marrow transplants, human Lassa virus transmission, viral hemorrhagic fever and other virulent diseases.

Strict Barrier Nursing

Strict barrier nursing, which is also known as "rigid barrier nursing", is used for the rarer and more specific deadly viruses and infections: smallpox, Ebola and rabies. Strict barrier nursing is a lot more demanding in terms of safety measure requirements because of the catastrophic effects that can occur if the disease or virus is allowed through the barrier. If patients cannot be isolated from one another completely, they have to at least be isolated from the rest of the patients within the hospital. In strict barrier nursing the patients and staff are usually isolated from the common population, and every attempt is made to establish a barrier between the inside and outside of the ward. The staff going on duty have to remove all outer clothing, pass through an airlock and put on a new set of PPE. When a staff member is going off duty, they are required to take a thorough shower and leave everything that was taken into the room to be disinfected or destroyed. While strict barrier nursing methods cannot always be enforced, especially in lower income areas and countries, any modifications made must be based on sound principles. Since infection can be spread through fomites, clothes or oxygen, all efforts must be made to limit the spread of these vessels. The doctor's or nurse's hands must be thoroughly washed after touching anything in the cubicle. Taps and door-handles should be elbow- or foot-operated. Hands should be washed in the cubicle and dried outside to eliminate contamination from paper or cloth towels. In addition, antiseptic hand-cream, dispensed from a foot-operated wall container would also serve as an additional precaution.

Psychiatric Effects of Barrier Nursing

Positive Effects

- Older patients and patients with more experience are content with their situation and approach it with more positivity.

- Some patients enjoy the experience of privacy and quietness that a single barrier room provided.

Negative Effects

- Barrier nursing/isolation influences the quality of care and opportunity for emotional support of the patient.

- Barrier nursing imposes barriers on the expression of a patient's own identity and any normal interpersonal relationships that he/she may have.

- Barrier nursing can lead to anxiety, anger, frustration and fear especially if the patient isn't given enough information, or incorrect information on their disease.

- Barrier nursing equipment can sometimes aggravate the social stigma associated with their infectious disease.

Although participants understood the importance for personalized protective equipment, they still found that its use increased their fear and sense of stigma.

- Placing patients in barrier nursing rooms may expose them to less medical care or access to associated treatment.

Solutions to Negative Effects of Barrier Nursing/Isolation

- Empowering patients with accurate and meaningful information about their disease as a means of coping with their experience.

- Providing accurate information for family and visitors in order to ensure or reduce their initial illinformed fear of becoming infected.

- Ensuring patients have access to a telephone as a means of communication with the outside world.

- Designing facilities with windows and free space that allow patients to see the outside world and mitigate their feelings of confinement.

Nursing Theory

In modern health care, nursing theories assist nurses by offering a number of different strategies and approaches to providing patients with optimal care. As today's nurse educators train the next generation of nurses, they are responsible for equipping future nurses with the key components of the foremost theories, so that these nurses can utilize the methods that best fit their patient care needs. The following five nursing theories are some of the leading approaches used, offering meaningful insights that accommodate each patient's individual health care needs and interests.

Leininger's Culture Care Theory

Believing that culture, together with care, is a powerful construct that is essential to health and prosperity, Madeleine Leininger founded the culture care theory during her long career as a certified nurse, administrator, author, educator, and public figure. Also referred to as the theory of transcultural nursing, the culture care theory addresses the care needs of patients of diverse cultures in hospitals, clinics, and other community settings. To help nurses and nurse educators develop realistic, new, and comprehensive care practices that effectively serve the unique cultural demands of the ill, Leininger structured the culture care theory with these four major tenets:

1. Though culture care practices are inherently diverse, there are some universal attributes and similarities that recur within the patterns and expressions of care.

2. Culture care is strongly influenced by relevant aspects of an individual's worldview, ethnic history, language, environmental context, and societal structure. These factors critically influence personal patterns that can be used to predict health, prosperity, sickness, and how someone behaves when confronted with difficult care concepts, like disability and death.

3. An individual's culture-based ideas of care, medicine, and health factors can greatly influence health outcomes.

4. There are three transcultural modes of action available to nursing care professionals:

   o Culture preservation and/or maintenance,

   o Culture accommodation and/or negotiation, and

   o Culture re-patterning and/or restructuring.

Humanistic Nursing Theory

This theory focuses on the human aspect of nursing and was developed by doctors Josephine Paterson and Loretta Zderad during the 1960s based on their interest in mixing nursing with phenomenological and existential philosophies. Paterson and Zderad were sure that, through examining their own individual experiences and personally connecting with patients, clinical nurses would be able to devise new theoretical arguments that could potentially become useful guides for other nursing care professionals. In order to focus on the overall human experience when caring for a patient, a nurse should treat the individual as being more than just a number—the nurse needs to connect with the patient in an interpersonal fashion to develop the best care strategy. This requires engaging in dialogue with the patient, so that the nurse may blend their personal and emotional perspectives with the patient's respective viewpoints in order to develop a well-rounded understanding of the medical situation. Through the following three concepts of humanistic nursing, nurse educators can help nurses learn how to effectively define themselves, their work, and their relationships with their patients and colleagues to ensure that their planned treatment strategies account for the personal and emotional viewpoints of every involved party:

- Dialogue – Establishing complete communicative relations in three different forms:

  o   Person to person dialogues,

  o   Person to object dialogues, and

  o   Group dialogues in the form of a community of two or more people.

- Community – Through community, two or more people are able to discover the innate meaning of their actions by sharing ideas and experiences with one another.

- Phenomenological Nursing – Intended to help nurses describe their experiences within the context of humanistic dialogue; phenomenological nursing has five phases:

  o   Preparing to understand experiences and perceptions, without prejudice and judgment, while acknowledging one's own personal worldview.

  o   Getting to know the other person's view on their experiences as a nurse or patient.

  o   Reflecting upon previous experiences to analyze, classify, and compare one's own experiences to that of another nurse or patient.

  o   Synthesizing the information gained through the first three phases, based on the realities of one's own worldview.

  o   Using the ideas that have been inferred from each situation now represented as a whole concept or theory that represents a nurse's understanding of their experiences or their patient's experiences.

Need Theory

Virginia Henderson, member of the American Nurses Association's Hall of Fame and recipient of the title of "Foremost Nurse of the 20th Century," dedicated her nursing career to aiding other nurses in formulating their own theories. Her most profound view of nursing can be found within the nursing need theory, which focuses on increasing a patient's personal independence while hospitalized for the purpose of expediting their recovery. By integrating Henderson's nursing need theory within their curricula, educators can teach nurses how to create practical therapeutic plans that supplement a patient's own strengths, allowing the patient to gradually become more independent and eventually regain their ability to care for themselves. The theory is broken down into 14 components that are categorized as physiological, psychological, spiritual, and social needs:

- Physiological needs cover areas relating to sleep, eating, dress and environment.
- Psychological needs highlight communication, emotion, learning and handling fears.
- Spiritual needs relate to faith and worship.
- Social needs cover accomplishment and recreational activities.

Self-care Nursing Theory

Dorothea Orem was a renowned American nursing theorist and educator who conceived the self-care nursing theory, which teaches nurses to assist patients in improving their ability to perform acts of self-care. Self-care, for the purpose of this theory, is defined as the practice of activities that individuals perform to maintain their personal health and well-being. To implement the self-care nursing theory effectively in their teachings, nursing educators must apply three interrelated theories:

- The Theory of Self-care – This theory is centered on identifying the universal basic self-care processes that most humans are usually capable of performing. Examples of these universal processes are taking in sufficient air, water, and nutrition, preventing exposure to hazards, and promoting development within social groups. As humans develop and encounter illness, injury, or disease, this list grows to include situation-specific self-care processes like seeking medical attention.

- The Self-care Deficit Theory – This theory focuses on situations where a person has become unable to perform continuous self-care. Orem coined these five methods of assisting patients who are unable to tend to their own self-care needs:

  o Taking action for the sake of the patient.

  o Providing patients with guidance.

  o Providing patients with support.

  o Providing patients with an environment that promotes personal development.

  o Teaching patients how to cope with obstacles they may potentially face in the future.

The Theory of Nursing Systems – Within this theory, three systems are used to identify a person's need for nursing care:

- Wholly Compensatory Nursing Systems – These systems support people who are entirely unable to care for themselves, and therefore, their well-being is entirely dependent on others.

- Partial Compensatory Nursing Systems – In this system, the nurse and patient each play some role in performing personal care.

- Supportive-Educative Nursing Systems – The patient is able to perform the necessary self-care activities, but needs active guidance from a nursing care professional.

Theory of Interpersonal Relations

Developed in 1952 by Hildegard Peplau, the interpersonal relations theory highlights the significance of a nurse and patient forming a productive partnership. Nurses become more effective at providing therapy to their patients and nursing them back to good health by building a relationship based on mutual respect for one another. Nursing educators can comprehensively teach their students this useful theory by relaying the following four phases:

1. Orientation – In the first phase, the nurse helps the patient become engaged with the treatment process by providing them with information and answering any questions.

2. Identification – This phase is entered once a patient begins expressing their feelings to the nurse, effectively decreasing the patient's feelings of helplessness.

3. Exploitation – At this point, the patient allows themselves to become more dependent, fully utilizing the services being offered by their nurse or other health care representatives.

4. Resolution – During the final phase, the nurse and patient work to dissolve any professional and therapeutic relationships that have formed, as the patient's need for nursing care has ended. This step is a critical aspect for a patient to maintain a healthy emotional balance.

Nursing Models

Nursing models are usually described as a representation of reality or a more simple way of organising a complex phenomenon. The nursing model is a consolidation of both concepts and the assumption that combine them into a meaningful arrangement. A model is a way of presenting a situation in such a way that it shows the logical terms in order to showcase the structure of the original idea. The term nursing model cannot be used interchangeably with nursing theory.

Components of Nursing Modeling

There are three main key components to a nursing model:

- Statement of goal that the nurse is trying to achieve.

- Set of beliefs and values.

- Awareness, skills and knowledge the nurse needs to practice.

The first important step in development of ideas about nursing is to establish the body approach essential to nursing, then to analyse the beliefs and values around those.

Common Concepts of Nursing Modeling: A Metaparadigm

A metaparadigm contains philosophical worldviews and concepts that are unique to a discipline and defines boundaries that separate it from other disciplines. A metaparadigm is intended to help guide others to conduct research and utilize the concepts for academia within that discipline. The nursing metaparadigm consist of four main concepts: person, health, environment, and nursing.

- The person (Patient)

- The environment

- Health

- Nursing (Goals, Roles Functions)

Each theory is regularly defined and described by a Nursing Theorist. The main focal point of nursing out of the four various common concepts is the person (patient).

Nursing Process

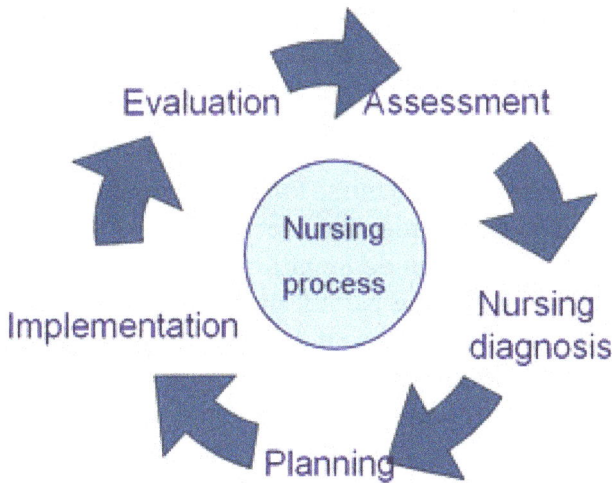

The nursing process is a scientific method used by nurses to ensure the quality of patient care. This approach can be broken down into five separate steps are mentioned below.

Assessment Phase

The first step of the nursing process is assessment. During this phase, the nurse gathers information about a patient's psychological, physiological, sociological, and spiritual status. This data can be collected in a variety of ways. Generally, nurses will conduct a patient interview. Physical examinations, referencing a patient's health history, obtaining a patient's family history, and general observation can also be used to gather assessment data. Patient interaction is generally the heaviest during this evaluative phase.

Diagnosing Phase

The diagnosing phase involves a nurse making an educated judgment about a potential or actual health problem with a patient. Multiple diagnoses are sometimes made for a single patient. These assessments not only include an actual description of the problem (e.g. sleep deprivation) but also whether or not a patient is at risk of developing further problems. These diagnoses are also used to determine a patient's readiness for health improvement and whether or not they may have developed a syndrome. The diagnoses phase is a critical step as it is used to determine the course of treatment.

Planning Phase

Once a patient and nurse agree on the diagnoses, a plan of action can be developed. If multiple diagnoses need to be addressed, the head nurse will prioritize each assessment and devote attention to severe symptoms and high risk factors. Each problem is assigned a clear, measurable goal for the expected beneficial outcome. For this phase, nurses generally refer to the evidence-based Nursing outcome classification, which is a set of standardized terms and measurements for tracking patient wellness. The Nursing interventions classification may also be used as a resource for planning.

Implementing Phase

The implementing phase is where the nurse follows through on the decided plan of action. This plan is specific to each patient and focuses on achievable outcomes. Actions involved in a nursing care plan include monitoring the patient for signs of change or improvement, directly caring for the patient or performing necessary medical tasks, educating and instructing the patient about further health management, and referring or contacting the patient for follow-up. Implementation can take place over the course of hours, days, weeks, or even months.

Evaluation Phase

Once all nursing intervention actions have taken place, the nurse completes an evaluation to determine of the goals for patient wellness have been met. The possible patient outcomes are generally described under three terms: patient's condition improved, patient's condition stabilized, and patient's condition deteriorated, died, or discharged. In the event the condition of the patient has shown no improvement, or if the wellness goals were not met, the nursing process begins again from the first step.

References

- Formenty, Pierre (2014). Emerging Infectious Diseases. Amsterdam: Academic Press. pp. 121–134. ISBN 9780124169753

- Health-care: businessdictionary.com, Retrieved 10 July 2018

- Gammon, J. (March 26 – April 8, 1998). "A review of the development of isolation precautions". British Journal of Nursing (Mark Allen Publishing). 7 (6): 307–310. doi:10.12968/bjon.1998.7.6.5727. ISSN 0966-0461. PMID 9661353

- Healthcare-primary-secondary-and-tertiary-brief-description: triotree.com, Retrieved 20 March 2018

- Kolcaba, Katherine (March–April 2001). "Evolution of the mid range theory of comfort for outcomes research". Nursing Outlook. 49: 86–92. doi:10.1067/mno.2001.110268 – via Elsevier

- Our-top-10-great-attributes-of-a-nurse-119857: diversitynursing.com, Retrieved 28 May 2018

- Chinn, Peggy; Kramer, Maeona (November 30, 2010). Integrated Theory & Knowledge Development in Nursing (8 ed.). St. Louis: Mosby. ISBN 0323077188

- Nursing-Process-Steps: nursingprocess.org, Retrieved 21 April 2018

- Martinsen, Elin Håkonsen (March 2011). "Care for Nurses Only? Medicine and the Perceiving Eye". Health Care Analysis. Berlin, Germany: Springer Science+Business Media. 19 (1): 15–27. doi:10.1007/s10728-010-0161-9. ISSN 1065-3058. PMC 3037482. PMID 21136173

Services Provided by Nurses

A nurse is an important health care professional who is entrusted with a number of resposibilities. These include bed management, bed-making, routine mouth care, morning care and respite care. These have been elaborately discussed in this chapter.

Bed Management

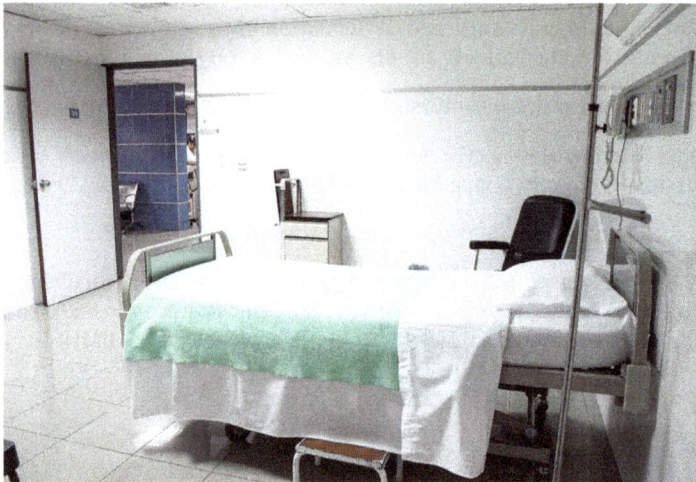

Hospital bed management is one of the most important tasks to enable the hospital to function as the performance of many hospital departments are dependent on the way the beds are managed. Bed management involves constantly monitoring hospital admissions, discharges and patient movement within the hospital so that accurate information is gathered to identify bed availability across all wards. The bed managers use this information to place patients in beds on the wards that are most appropriate to their needs. Bed management is an important task of nurses.

Bed-making

Bed making is one of the important nursing techniques to prepare various types of bed for patients or clients to ensure comfort and useful position for a particular condition.

The bed is especially important for patients who are sick. The nurse plays inevitable role to ensure comfort and cleanliness for ill patient. It should be adaptable to various positions as per patient's need because they spend varying amount of the day in bed.

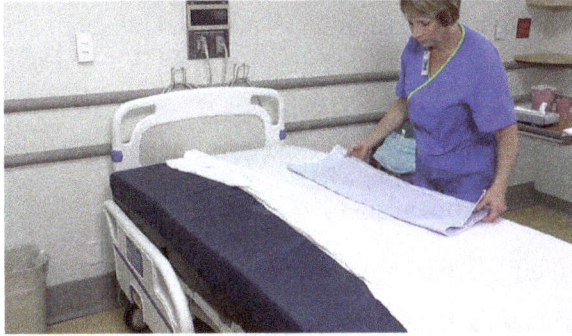

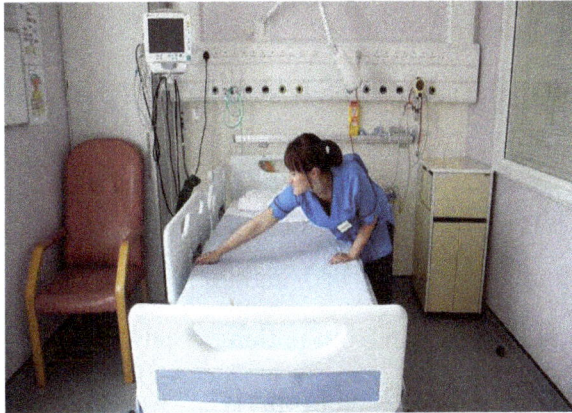

Types of Bed Making in Hospital

Nursing staff make different types of bed according to patient condition those are listed below:

1. Simple bed or unoccupied bed

    o   Close bed (Admission bed),

    o   Open bed.

2. Occupied bed,

3. Cardiac bed,

4. Fowler's bed,

5. Fracture bed,

6. Operation bed.

Purpose of Bed Making in Hospital:

Bed-making is a nursing art. The purpose of the bed-making should be patients or clients-centered. The main purposes of bed-making are to prevent complications by ensuring comfort and security to patient.

1. To provide rest and sleep.

2. To provide physical and psychological comfort and security to the patient.

3. To give the unit neat appearance.

4. To establish an effective nurse patients relationship.

5. To provide active and passive exercise to the patient.

6. To promote fresh and cleanliness.

7. To develop skill in the posture/body alignment of the nurse in bed-making.

8. To observe, identify and prevent patient's complications.

9. To accommodate the patient's needs.

10. To reduce patient's exertion by bed-making.

11. To eliminate irritants to skin from patient's body.

12. To dispose soiled and dirty linen properly.

13. Another purpose of bed-making is to save time, effort and material properly.

Basic Principle of Bed Making in Hospital

Skillful bed making contributes patients comfort. Some basic principles of bed-making are pointed below:

1. It is important to learn that how to make a bed in such a way where least amount of energy and time is required.

2. During bed-making, use good body movement and make each step purposeful.

3. Keep everything ready on bed side before starting bed-making.

4. Change bed linen frequently to assure cleanliness.

5. To ensure the patient need by providing a safe and comfortable bed.

6. It should have a finished appearance.

7. To make bed tight and free from wrinkles, place all linen straight line on the bed.

8. Prevent complications of prolonged bed ridden patient such as pressure sore.

9. Soiled linen or linen whether clean or dirty should not be thrown on the floor, but it is should be kept in a dirty linen box.

10. After cleaning bed, dump soap water and disinfectant properly.

11. Try to prevent cross infection of microorganism during bed making.

12. Ensure all bed making in a nursing unit alike for uniformity of appearance.

Things to keep in Mind during Bed Making in Hospitals

During bed-making we should remember some knowledge those are useful for us and also to patient.

1. During bed-making, bed position keep elevated and ensures nursing staff's good body alignments.

2. During the procedure, the nurse should study her movements so as to avoid waste of time and energy.

3. After completing, bed should be lower position.

4. During occupied bed making, confirm patient safety and comfort.

5. Wash hands before and after bed making and use gloves during bed-making.

6. Maintain privacy while making bed.

7. Keep soiled linen away from uniform which may have germs.

8. Do not shake dirty linen to prevent germs spread around room.

9. Do not mix soiled and clean linen during bed-making.

10. For bed ridden patient, mattress must be turned air and ensure free of lumps and fold.

Changing Bed Sheets

Setting up the Bedding

Ideally, you should change bed sheets when a bed is empty. However, if a person is on bed rest and is either not supposed to or is unable to get out of bed, you'll need to change the sheets while the bed is occupied. This process can be strenuous for the person occupying the bed, so make sure your supplies are ready beforehand to stream-line the process as much as possible. For patients experiencing pain, give a prescribed PRN analgesic thirty to sixty minutes before you change the bed linens. An occupied bed is usually changed after a bed bath.

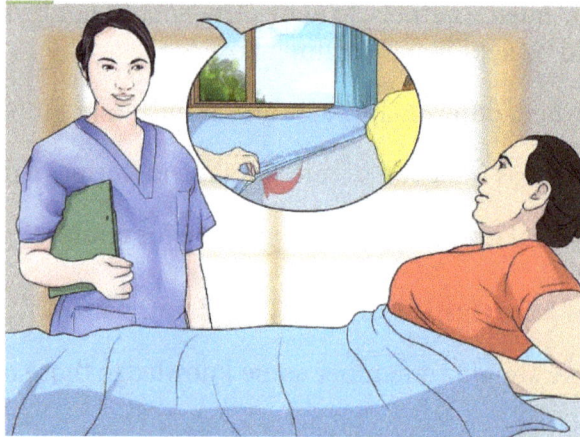

1. Tell the patient what you're doing: Knock on the door before entering the room. Whether or not you think the patient can hear you, explain what you're doing and make sure that you provide privacy for the patient. Close the blinds or curtains of any window as well as the patient's privacy curtain. Introduce yourself and greet the patient using their name.

- Try saying, "Hello, [patient name]! My name is [your name] and I'm the CNA who will be changing your sheets today. First I'll wash my hands, and prepare the supplies. I'll be right back, okay?"

- If the patient is sitting upright, ask if it is alright that you lay them down flat.

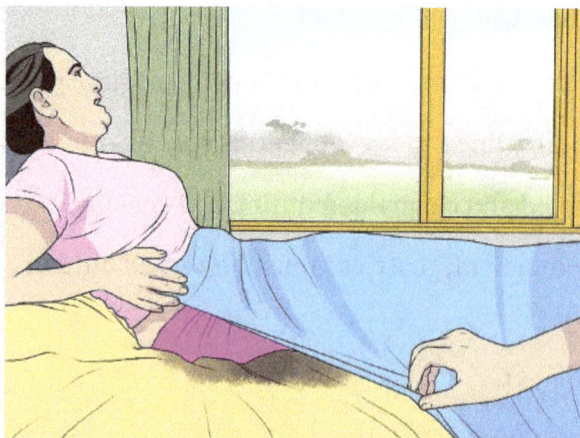

2. Check the state of the linens: You may not have to replace all the bedding every day. However, you may need to change the bottom and top sheets and the pillowcase regu-larly. The mattress pad, bedspread and blanket can remain if they are dry and unsoiled.

- Bedding that is at all dirty or wet from urine, stool, blood, emesis or perspiration should be changed.

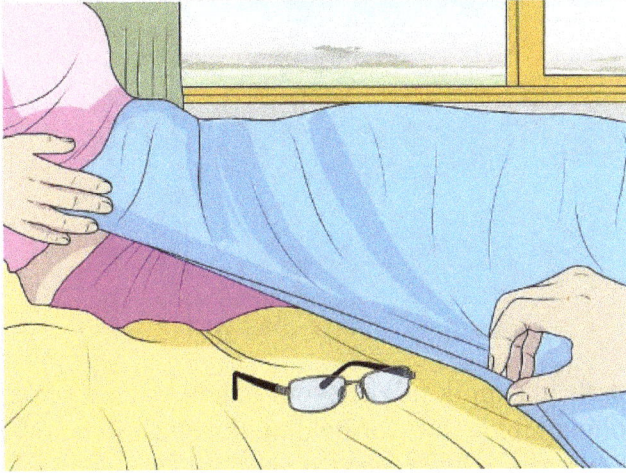

3. Check the bedding for items: Make sure there are no hearing aids, dentures, jewelry, glasses, tissues or other items in the bed before changing the linens. This way you will be able to remove soiled sheets without shaking them.

- Make sure no tubes are tangled in the bed sheets.

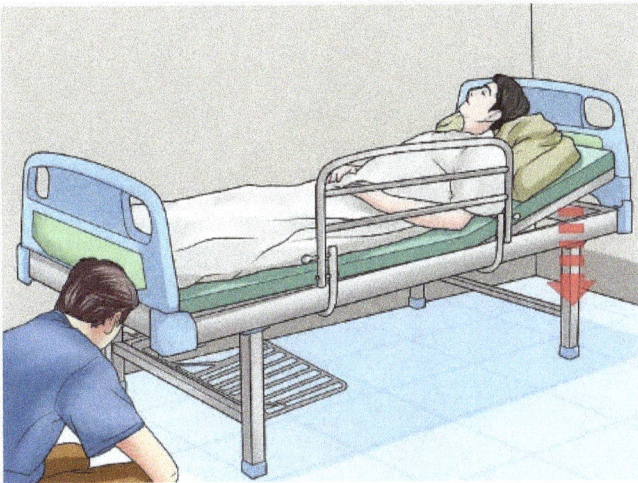

4. Adjust the bed: Put the bed at a comfortable height, and flat if possible. Ensure that you won't have to stretch or bend over the bed in order to replace the bedding. Put the side rails up so the occupant won't roll out and will have something to grasp onto.

- If the bed does not have side rails, you will need two people for this process: one for making the bed and the other for holding the patient securely on the bed.

- If there are wheels on the bed, make sure that they are locked.

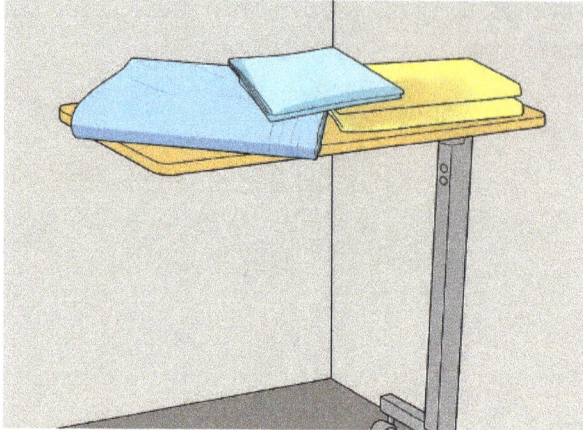

5. Create an area for clean supplies: Wash your hands and put on gloves. Have a clean surface such as a rolling table ready for holding the clean items. You can also use the over bed table as a work area. Only touch the supplies with clean hands.

- Put the clean items you need on the clean area. For example, a flat sheet, fitted sheet, and a pillow case. Also include a clean privacy blanket, and a draw sheet if desired.

Changing the Sheets

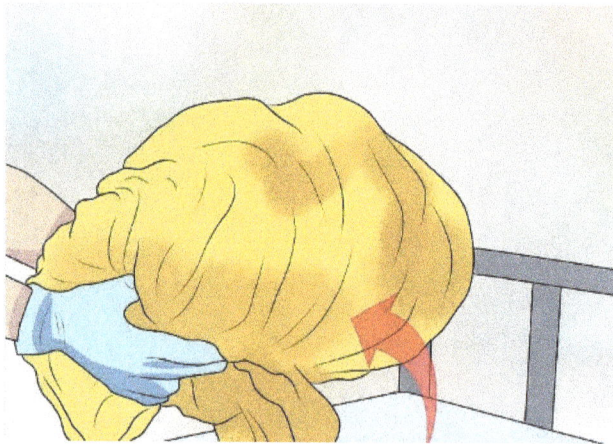

1. Remove soiled items: Hold soiled linens away from your clothing when transferring them to a hamper. Don't shake the linens, as this can introduce micro-organisms into the air. If the clean linens accidentally touch the floor, put them in the dirty hamper and get new clean sheets.

- Don't allow soiled linens to touch your face or uniform.

- If a hamper is not immediately available, place soiled sheets in a plastic bag or laundry basket. Never place them on the nightstand or floor, even temporarily.

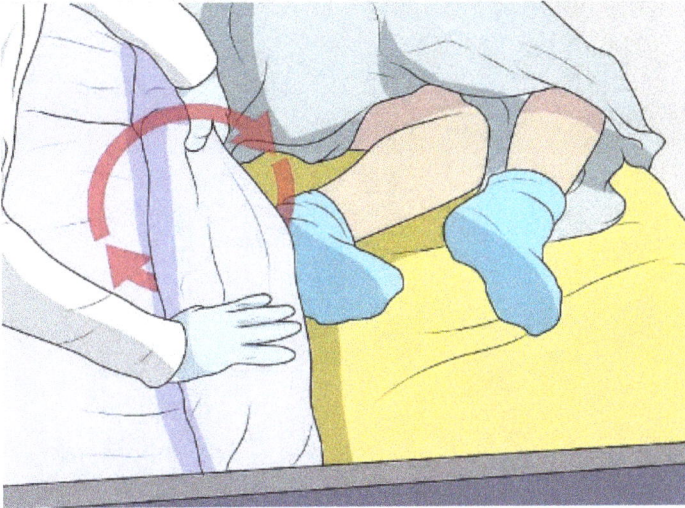

2. Change the fitted sheet: Gently roll the patient onto their side. Remove the fitted sheet by rolling it towards the patient. Put a pad where the patient's hips will lie. Then roll a clean linen towards you. Carefully roll the patient onto the clean linen.

- Tuck the corners and sides of the clean fitted sheet neatly under the mattress. Pull the clean linen tightly on the bed so that it's wrinkle-free.

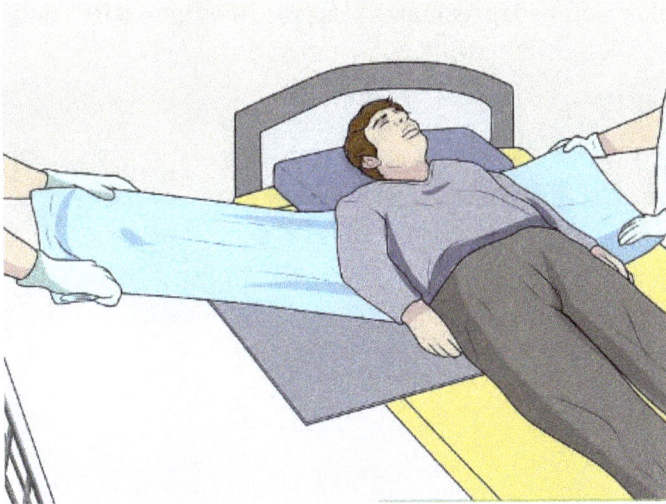

3. Use a draw sheet if you're working with a partner: This will allow you to move the patient from side to side during the process. Fold a sheet in half and stretch it across the middle of the bed to use for this purpose. Place the draw sheet on top of the bottom sheet, from the patient's shoulders to buttocks with at least six inches of sheet left on each side.

- Pulling the sheet on with a helper permits you to move even a large onto their side or higher up on the mattress. If you need a demonstration, ask an OT or PT.

Changing the Remaining Linens

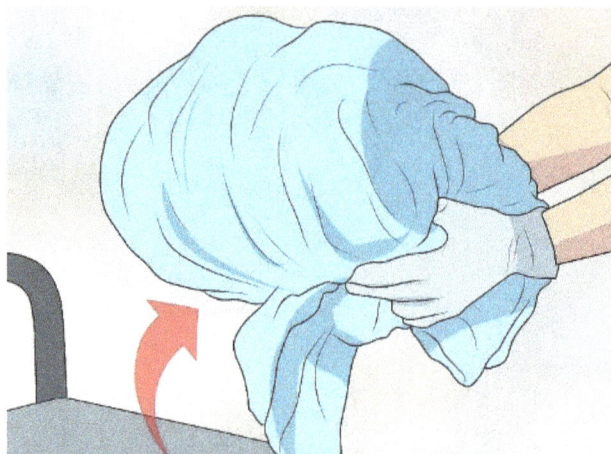

1. Remove the top bedding: Place a privacy blanket over the patient. Loosen the top bedding at the end of the bed. Fold the bedspread to the foot of the bed and take it away by holding it at the center. Repeat with the blanket.

- Only put the bedrail down on the side you're working on. Never step away from the bed at all when the side rail is down.

- If the blanket and bedspread are dirty, replace them with clean ones. Otherwise place them over a chair while you change the sheets.

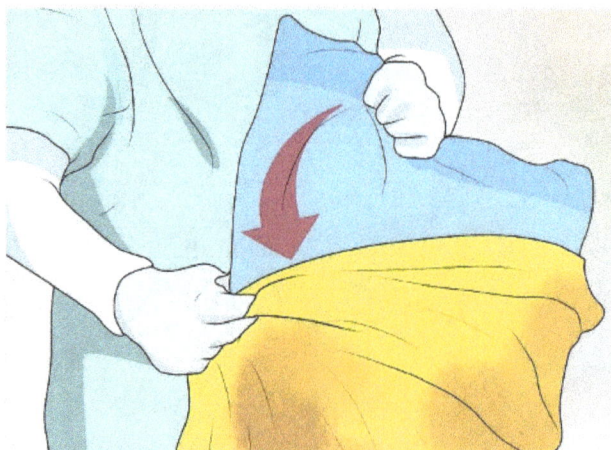

2. Remove the dirty pillowcase: Support the person's head and neck as you remove the pillow. Gently rest the patient's head back down on the bed. Remove the dirty pillowcase by unrolling it away from you. Put the pillowcase in the laundry hamper. Change your gloves to a clean pair.

- Try saying, "I'm going to use my hands to gently support your head and neck as I remove the pillow now, so that I can put on a fresh pillowcase for you."

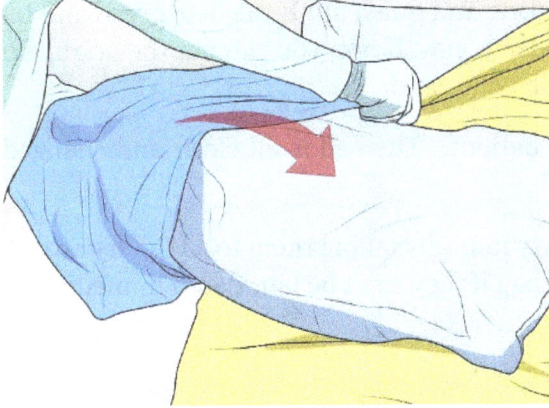

3. Put on a fresh pillowcase: Put the clean pillowcase over your hand and arm so that you can grasp the center of the pillow with your covered hand. Unroll the clean pillowcase onto the pillow. Carefully lift the patient's head and neck and put the pillow with the clean pillowcase on it under their head.

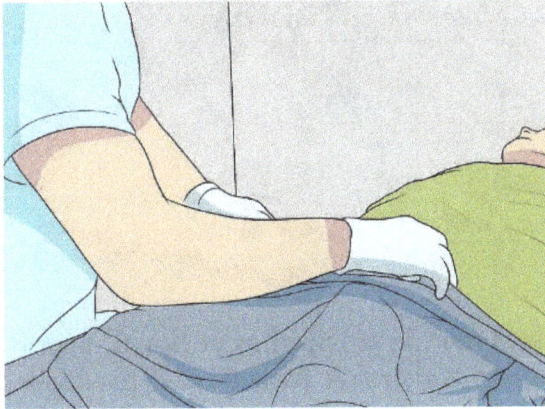

4. Cover the patient. Put a clean flat sheet and a blanket over the patient. Secure the lower corners of the sheet with mitered corners. Move the occupant into a comfortable resting position and adjust the bedding as needed.

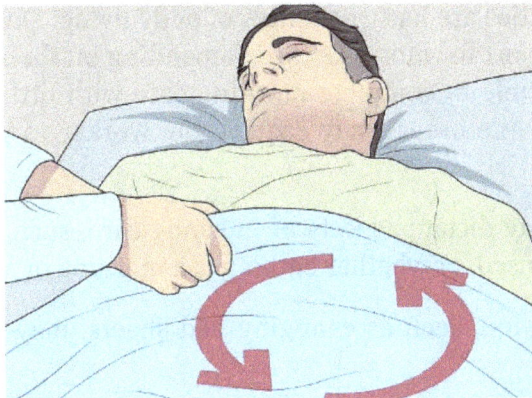

5. Replace the top blankets and finish up: If the bedspread and blanket were soiled, replace them with new, clean ones. If not, you can put the original ones back on. Dispose of your gloves and wash your hands.

- Try telling the patient, "The bed is all clean and changed now. Thank you for your patience."

- Remove the dirty items by taking them to a laundry area. Keep them in a plastic bag or laundry bag if they can't be laundered immediately.

Morning Care

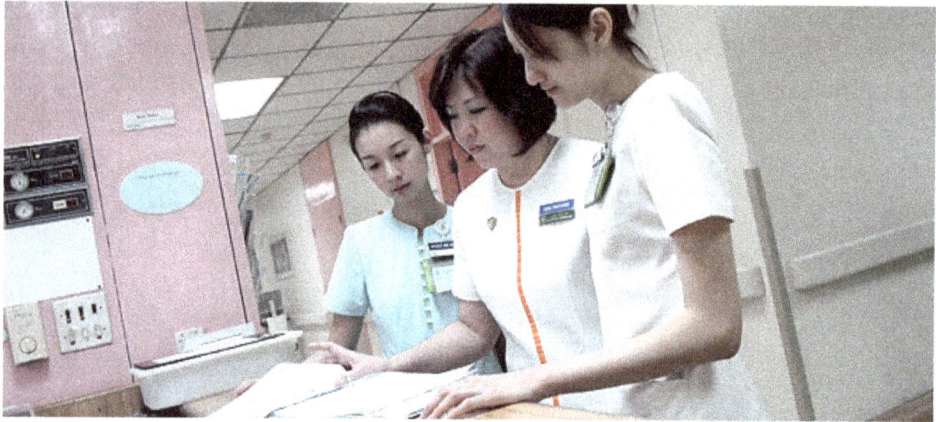

Morning care is a hygiene routine provided by personal support workers, nursing assistants, nurses, and other workers for patients and residents of care facilities each morning. The care routine typically includes washing the face, combing hair, shaving, putting on cosmetics, toileting, getting dressed, and similar activities. Nurses may also check the patients' temperature, check medical equipment, replenish IV bags, change dressings, or do other daily or semi-daily tasks at this time.

Most morning care duties are basic activities of daily living. Different people require different levels of support for morning care, depending on their performance status. Some people may be able to complete morning care with little or no support from healthcare workers, while others may require the worker to perform all the tasks completely.

Patient preferences may dictate aspects of morning care, such as the order of tasks done, the type of soap used, or whether bathing is a morning or afternoon activity.

Some basic housekeeping, such as changing bed sheets, may be done at the same time.

Respite Care

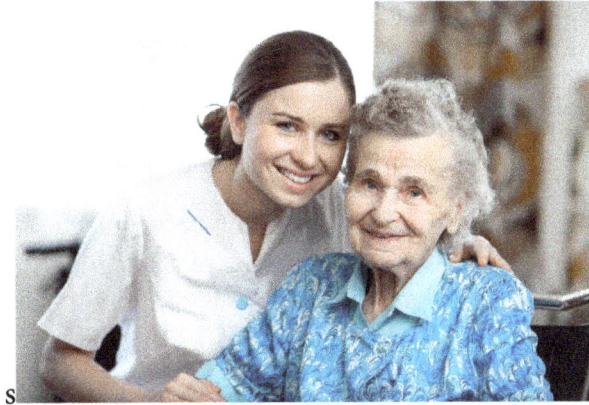

Respite care is planned or emergency temporary care provided to caregivers of a child or adult.

Respite programs provide planned short-term and time-limited breaks for families and other unpaid care givers of children with a developmental delay, children with behavioral problems, adults with an intellectual disability, and adults with cognitive loss in order to support and maintain the primary care giving relationship. Respite also provides a positive experience for the person receiving care. The term "short break" is used in some countries to describe respite care.

Even though many families take great joy in providing care to their loved ones so that they can remain at home, the physical, emotional and financial consequences for the family caregiver can be overwhelming without some support, such as respite. Respite provides a break for the family caregiver, which may prove beneficial to the health of the caregiver. 60% of family caregivers age 19-64 surveyed recently by the Commonwealth Fund reported fair or poor health, one or more chronic conditions, or a disability, compared with only 33% of non caregivers.

Respite has been shown to help sustain family caregiver health and well being, avoid or delay out-of-home placements, and reduce the likelihood of abuse and neglect. An outcome based evaluation pilot study showed that respite may also reduce the likelihood of divorce and help sustain marriages.

Respite care or respite services are also a family support service, and in the US is a long-term services and support (LTSS) as described by the Consortium of Citizens with Disabilities in Washington, DC as of 2013.

Models for Respite Care

There are various models for providing respite care.

In-home Respite

In-home care is popular for obvious reasons. The temporary caregiver comes to the regular care receiver's home, and gets to know the care receiver in his or her normal environment. The temporary caregiver learns the family routine, where medicines are stored, and the care receiver is not inconvenienced by transportation and strange environments. In this model, friends, relatives and paid professionals may be used. Depending on the state, Medicaid or Medicare may be used to help cover costs.

Respite (In-home) Services means intermittent or regularly scheduled temporary non-medical care (which can be health care financed) and/or supervision provided in the person's home. In-home Respite services are support services which typically include:

- Assisting the family members to enable a person with developmental disabilities to stay at home.

- Providing appropriate care and supervision to protect that person's safety in the absence of a family member.

- Relieving family members from the constantly demanding responsibility of providing care.

- Attending to basic self-help needs and other activities that would ordinarily be performed by the family member.

Respite (Out-of-home) Services

Respite services are provided in the community at diverse sites, and by service providers which operate licensed residential facilities or bill under a category called respite.

Respite services typically are obtained from a respite vendor, by use of vouchers and/or alternative respite options. Vouchers are a means by which a family may choose their own service provider directly through a payment, coupon or other type of authorization. For more information about respite services contact your regional center representative.

Respite and Community

Respite is an early service from the 1950s in which parents sought funding from the government for payments for specialized childcare, called respite provided by the parent organizations themselves. Professional models of respite developed in the 1970s included community recreation options for the adults (e.g., at Ys, neighborhood centers, run and walks) as the parents had a "respite" or break from care giving. The state of New York has over 950 service providers in intellectual disabilities alone as of the mid-2000s.

Group Homes and Respite

Many parents wished to have a designated facility to drop off their child for "respite" (e.g., weekend), which in institutional days is a role state governments played before it was recognized that the child had rights of their own. States did fund and develop community respite centers (small homes), and also designate places in group homes for respite, including innovative friends of the home in conjunction with the private, non-profit sector.

Specialized Facility

Another model uses a specialized, local facility where the care receiver may stay for a few days or a few weeks. The advantage of this model is that the specialized facility will probably have better access to emergency facilities and professional assistance if needed.

Emergency Respite

There may be the need for respite care on an emergency basis. When using "planned" emergency care, the caregiver has already identified a provider or facility to call in case there is an emergency. Many homecare agencies, adult day care, health centers, and residential care facilities provide emergency respite care.

Sitter-companion Services

Sitter-companion services are one of about 6 different innovative community approaches or models to respite care which were developed internationally. They are all paid services in the US, which are only available to designated "clients" of the service systems.

They are sometimes provided by local civic groups, the faith community and other community organizations. A regular sitter-companion can provide friendly respite care for a few hours, once or twice a week. Care must be taken to assure that the sitter-companion is trained in what to do if an emergency occurs while the regular care-giver is out of the home.

Therapeutic Adult Day Care

Therapeutic adult daycare may provide respite care during business hours five days a week. However, in some instances, this care may also be provided 24 hours a day. Usually, these are facilities for designated clients only, and not related to family support services other than any specialized service is considered a family support to the family which desires it. However, this group is involved in also trying to re-institutionalize children which they also term a support to the parents as do the parents involved.

Routine Mouth Care

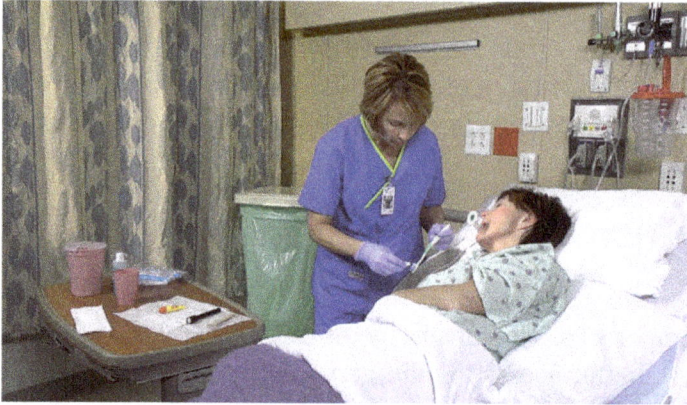

Mouth care should be given at least every morning and evening to all patients, and preferably after every meal. Routine mouth care is essentially assisting a patient to brush his teeth and to rinse his mouth thoroughly, as often as needed. The purposes are to keep the mouth clean, to prevent sores and mouth odors, to retard or prevent deterioration of teeth, and to refresh the patient.

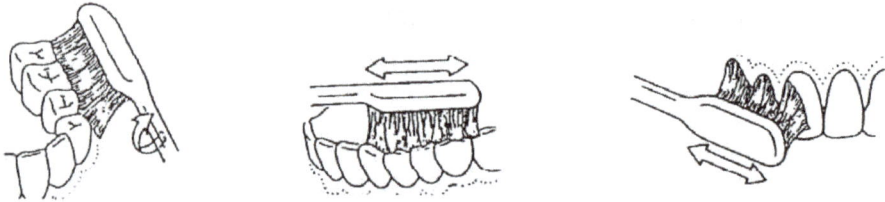

Cleaning the teeth

Equipment

The following equipment is appropriate for routine mouth care:

1. Glass of water.

2. Drinking tube if necessary.

3. Hand towel.

4. Toothbrush and dentifrice.

5. Mouthwash, if desired.

Procedure for Patient able to help Himself

Following is the procedure for routine mouth care for a bed patient able to help himself:

1. Place the patient in a comfortable position.

2. Arrange the equipment within his reach on the bedside cabinet or on an over bed table.

3. Remove and clean the equipment promptly when he is finished.

Rinse the toothbrush thoroughly under running water and allow it to air dry–not place the damp brush in the cabinet.

Procedure for a Patient Requiring Assistance

Following is the procedure for routine mouth care for a bed patient requiring some assistance:

1. Turn the patient on his side or if on his back, turn his head to the side.

2. Place a towel under his chin and over the bedding.

3. Pour the water over the brush; place dentifrice on it.

4. Give the patient his brush and hold the basin under his chin while he brushes his teeth.

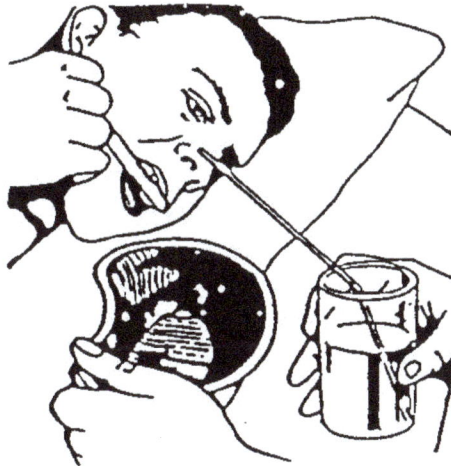

Assisting patient with mouth care.

5. Encourage the patient to rinse his mouth frequently, using the drinking tube, if necessary to draw water in his mouth. The basin receives the used rinse water.

6. Remove the basin; wipe his face and lips with the hand towel.

7. Remove and clean the equipment.

8. Wash your hands.

Procedure for a Patient unable to Brush his Teeth

Following is the procedure for providing mouth care for a patient unable to brush his teeth:

1. Proceed as in paragraph above except that all steps are done for the patient.

2. Finish the mouth cleansing with a gentle brushing of the tongue from back to front, and with a thorough final rinsing.

3. The patient's teeth should be flossed at least weekly.

References

- Carter, Pamela J. (2007-06-01). Lippincott's Textbook for Nursing Assistants: A Humanistic Approach to Caregiving. Lippincott Williams & Wilkins. p. 328. ISBN 9780781766852

- Bed-management-team, acute-care-services: iow.nhs.uk, Retrieved 28 March 2018

- Bed-making-nursing-purpose-principles: nursingexercise.com, Retrieved 11 May 2018

- Change-Sheets-in-an-Occupied-Bed: wikihow.com, Retrieved 24 June 2018

- 1-12-routine-mouth-care, lesson-1-hygiene-and-care-of-the-patient, basic-patient-care: brookside-press.org, Retrieved 22 June 2018

General Assessment

The gathering of informtion pertaining to a patient's physiological, sociological, psychological and spiritual health by a registered nurse is referred to as general assessment. All the diverse aspects related to the types and techniques of nursing assessment have been carefully analyzed in this chapter.

Nursing Assessment

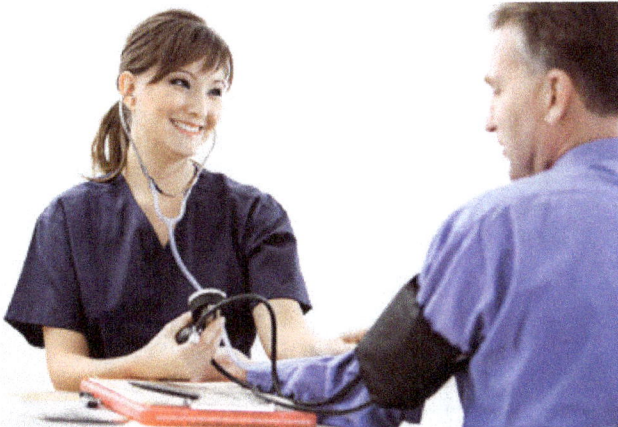

Assessment is a key component of nursing practice, required for planning and provision of patient and family centred care. Nursing assessment is the gathering of information about a patient's physiological, psychological, sociological, and spiritual status by a licensed Registered Nurse. It is the first step of the nursing process.

Principles

In planning and performing health assessment, the nurse needs to consider the following:

1. An accurate and timely health assessment provides foundation for nursing care and intervention.

2. A comprehensive assessment incorporates information about a client's physiologic, psychosocial, spiritual health, cultural and environmental factors as well as client's developmental status.

3. The health assessment process should include data collection, documentation and evaluation of the client's health status and responses to health problems and intervention.

4. All documentation should be objective, accurate, clear, concise, specific and current.

5. Health assessment is practised in all healthcare settings whenever there is nurse-client interaction.

6. Information gathered from health assessment should be communicated to other health care professionals in order to facilitate collaborative management of clients and for continuity of care.

7. Client's confidentiality should be kept.

Nursing Diagnosis

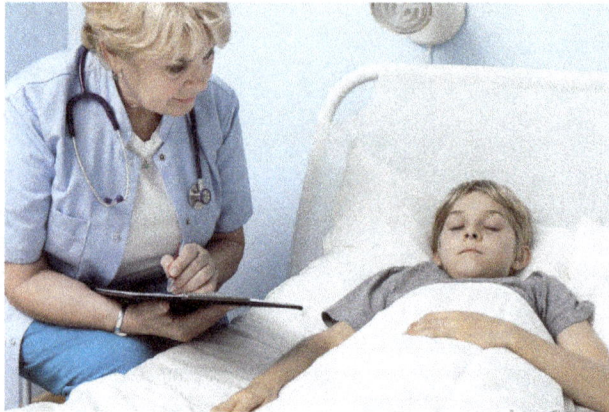

A nursing diagnosis is a clinical judgment concerning a human response to health conditions/life processes, or a vulnerability for that response, by an individual, family, group or community. A nursing diagnosis provides the basis for selection of nursing interventions to achieve outcomes for which the nurse has accountability.

Problem-focused Nursing Diagnosis

A clinical judgment concerning an undesirable human response to health conditions/life processes that exists in an individual, family, group, or community. In order to make a problem-focused diagnosis, the following must be present: defining characteristics (manifestations, signs, and symptoms) that cluster in patterns of related cues or inferences. Related factors (etiological factors) that are related to, contribute to, or antecedent to the diagnostic focus are also required.

Health-promotion Nursing Diagnosis

A clinical judgment concerning motivation and desire to increase well-being and to actualize human health potential. These responses are expressed by a readiness to enhance specific health behaviors, and can be used in any health state. Health promotion responses may exist in an individual, family, group, or community. In order to make a health-promotion diagnosis, the following must be present: defining characteristics which begin with the phrase, "Expresses desire to enhance...".

Risk Nursing Diagnosis

A clinical judgment concerning the vulnerability of an individual, family, group, or community for developing an undesirable human response to health conditions/life processes. In order to make a risk-focused diagnosis, the following must be present, supported by risk factors that contribute to increased vulnerability.

Syndrome

A clinical judgment concerning a specific cluster of nursing diagnoses that occur together, and are best addressed together and through similar interventions.In order to make a syndrome diagnosis, the following must be present: two or more nursing diagnoses must be used as defining characteristics. Related factors may be used if they add clarity to the definition, but are not required.

Diagnostic Axes

Axis

An axis is operationally defined as a dimension of the human response that is considered in the diagnostic process. There are seven axes which parallel the International Standards Reference Model for a Nursing Diagnosis:

- Axis 1: the diagnostic focus
- Axis 2: subject of the diagnosis (individual, caregiver, family, group, community)
- Axis 3: judgment (impaired, ineffective, etc.)
- Axis 4: location (bladder, auditory, cerebral, etc.)
- Axis 5: age (infant, child, adult, etc.)
- Axis 6: time (chronic, acute, intermittent)
- Axis 7: status of the diagnosis (problem-focused, risk, health promotion).

The axes are represented in the labels of the nursing diagnoses through their values. In some cases, they are named explicitly, such as with the diagnoses, Ineffective

Community Coping and Compromised Family Coping, in which the subject of the diagnosis (in the first instance "community" and in the second instance "family") is named using the two values "community" and "family" taken from Axis 2 (subject of the diagnosis). "Ineffective" and "compromised" are two of the values contained in Axis 3 (judgment).

In some cases, the axis is implicit, as is the case with the diagnosis, Activity intolerance, in which the subject of the diagnosis (Axis 2) is always the patient. In some instances an axis may not be pertinent to a particular diagnosis and therefore is not part of the nursing diagnostic label. For example, the time axis may not be relevant to every diagnosis. In the case of diagnoses without explicit identification of the subject of the diagnosis, it may be helpful to remember that NANDA-I defines patient as: "an individual, family, group or community".

Axis 1 (the diagnostic focus) and Axis 3 (judgment) are essential components of a nursing diagnosis. In some cases, however, the diagnostic focus contains the judgment (for example, Nausea); in these cases the judgment is not explicitly separated out in the diagnostic label. Axis 2 (subject of the diagnosis) is also essential, although, as described above, it may be implied and therefore not included in the label. The Diagnosis Development Committee requires these axes for submission; the other axes may be used where relevant for clarity.

Definitions of the Axes

Axis 1: The Diagnostic Focus

The diagnostic focus is the principal element or the fundamental and essential part, the root, of the diagnostic concept. It describes the "human response" that is the core of the diagnosis.

The diagnostic focus may consist of one or more nouns. When more than one noun is used (for example, Activity intolerance), each one contributes a unique meaning to the diagnostic focus, as if the two were a single noun; the meaning of the combined term, however, is different from when the nouns are stated separately. Frequently, an adjective (Spiritual) may be used with a noun (Distress) to denote the diagnostic focus Spiritual Distress.

Axis 2: Subject of the Diagnosis

The person(s) for whom a nursing diagnosis is determined. The values in Axis 2 which represent the NANDA-I definition of "patient" are:

- Individual: a single human being distinct from others, a person.

- Caregiver: a family member or helper who regularly looks after a child or a sick, elderly, or disabled person.

- Family: two or more people having continuous or sustained relationships, perceiving reciprocal obligations, sensing common meaning, and sharing certain obligations toward others; related by blood and/or choice.

- Group: a number of people with shared characteristics.

- Community: a group of people living in the same locale under the same governance. Examples include neighborhoods and cities.

Axis 3: Judgment

A descriptor or modifier that limits or specifies the meaning of the diagnostic focus. The diagnostic focus together with the nurse's judgment about it forms the diagnosis.

Axis 4: Location

Describes the parts/regions of the body and/or their related functions – all tissues, organs, anatomical sites, or structures.

Axis 5: Age

Refers to the age of the person who is the subject of the diagnosis (Axis 2). The values in Axis 5 are noted below, with all definitions except that of older adult being drawn from the World Health Organization (2013):

- Fetus: an unborn human more than eight weeks after conception, until birth

- Neonate: a child < 28 days of age

- Infant: a child > 28 days and <1 year of age

- Child: person aged 1 to 9 years, inclusive

- Adolescent: person aged 10 to 19 years, inclusive

- Adult: a person older than 19 years of age unless national law defines a person as being an adult at an earlier age

- Older adult: a person > 65 years of age.

Axis 6: Time

Describes the duration of the diagnostic concept (Axis 1). The values in Axis 6 are:

- Acute: lasting <3 months

- Chronic: lasting >3 months

- Intermittent: stopping or starting again at intervals, periodic, cyclic

- Continuous: uninterrupted, going on without stop.

Axis 7: Status of the Diagnosis

Refers to the actuality or potentiality of the problem/syndrome or to the categorization of the diagnosis as a health promotion diagnosis. The values in Axis 7 are: Problem-focused, Health Promotion, Risk, and Syndrome.

Process

The diagnositic process requires a nurse to use critical thinking. In addition to knowing the nursing diagnoses and their definitions, the nurse becomes aware of defining characteristics and behaviors of the diagnoses, related factors to the diagnoses, and the interventions suited for treating the diagnoses.

1. Assessment

   The first step of the nursing process is assessment. During this phase, the nurse gathers information about a patients psychological, physiological, sociological, and spiritual status. This data can be collected in a variety of ways. Generally, nurses will conduct a patient interview. Physical examinations, referencing a patient's health history, obtaining a patient's family history, and general observation can also be used to gather assessment data. Patient interaction is generally the heaviest during this evaluative stage.

2. Diagnosis

   The diagnosing phase involves a nurse making an educated judgement about a potential or actual health problem with a patient. Multiple diagnoses are sometimes made for a single patient. These assessments not only include a description of the problem or illness (e.g. sleep deprivation) but also whether or not a patient is at risk of developing further problems. These diagnoses are also used to determine a patient's readiness for health improvement and whether or not they may have developed a syndrome. The diagnoses phase is a critical step as it is used to determine the course of treatment.

3. Planning

   Once a patient and nurse agree of the diagnoses, a plan of action can be developed. If multiple diagnoses need to be addressed, the head nurse will prioritise each assessment and devote attention to severe symptoms and high risk patients. Each problem is assigned a clear, measurable goal for the expected beneficial outcome. For this phase, nurses generally refer to the evidence-based Nursing Outcome Classification, which is a set of standardised terms and measurements for tracking patient wellness. The Nursing Interventions Classification may also be used as a resource for planning.

4. Implementation

   The implementing phase is where the nurse follows through on the decided plan of action. This plan is specific to each patient and focuses on achievable outcomes. Actions involved in a nursing care plan include monitoring the patient for signs of change or improvement, directly caring for the patient or performing necessary medical tasks, educating and instructing the patient about further health management, and referring or contacting the patient for a follow-up. Implementation can take place over the course of hours, days, weeks, or even months.

5. Evaluation

   Once all nursing intervention actions have taken place, the nurse completes an evaluation to determine if the goals for patient wellness have been met. The possible patient outcomes are generally described under three terms: patient;s condition improved, patient's condition stabilised, and patient's condition deteriorated. In the event where the condition of the patient has shown no improvement, or if the wellness goals were not met, the nursing process begins again from the first step.

Examples

The following are nursing diagnoses arising from the nursing literature with varying degrees of authentication by ICNP or NANDA-I standards:

- Anxiety

- Constipation

- Pain

- Activity Intolerance

- Impaired Gas Exchange

- Excessive Fluid Volume

- Caregiver Role Strain

- Ineffective Coping

- Readiness for Enhanced Health Maintenance

- Readiness for enhanced spiritual well-being.

Types of Nursing Assessment

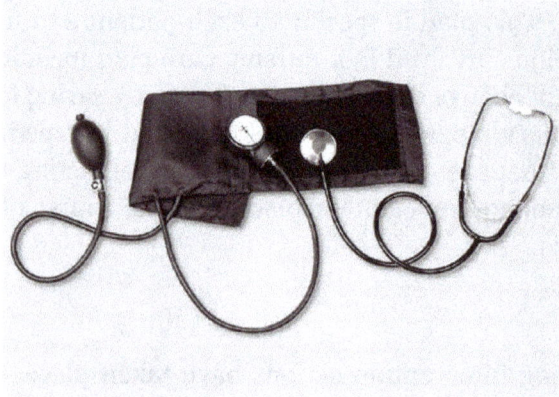

In general, there are four fundamental types of assessments that nurses perform:

- A comprehensive or complete health assessment

- An interval or abbreviated assessment

- A problem-focused assessment

- An assessment for special populations.

A comprehensive or complete health assessment usually begins with obtaining a thorough health history and physical exam. This type of assessment is usually performed in acute care settings upon admission, once your patient is stable, or when a new patient presents to an outpatient clinic.

If the patient has been under your care for some time, a complete health history is usually not indicated. Nurses perform an interval or abbreviated assessment at this time. These assessments are usually performed at subsequent visits in an outpatient setting, at change of shift, when returning from tests, or upon transfer to your unit from another in-house unit. This type of assessment is not as detailed as the complete assessment that occurs at admission. The advantage of an abbreviated assessment is that it allows you to thoroughly assess your patient in a shorter period of time.

The third type of assessment that you may perform is a problem-focused assessment. The problem-focused assessment is usually indicated after a comprehensive assessment has identified a potential health problem. The problem-focused assessment is also indicated when an interval or abbreviated assessment shows a change in status from the most current previous assessment or report you received, when a new symptom emerges, or the patient develops any distress. An advantage of the focused assessment is that it directs you to ask about symptoms and move quickly to conducting a focused physical exam.

The fourth type of assessment is the assessment for special populations, including:

- Pregnant patients

- Infants

- Children

- The elderly.

If there is any indication to perform a problem-focused or special population assessment during the comprehensive assessment, the assessment should occur after obtaining a baseline comprehensive assessment. Based upon the results of the problem-focused or special population assessment, you can decide how often to perform interval assessments to monitor your patient's identified problem.

The special assessment should not replace the comprehensive or interval assessments, but should augment both the complete and interval assessments. These will not be specifically addressed in this course. A systematic physical assessment remains one of the most vital components of patient care. A thorough physical assessment can be completed within a time frame that is practical and should never be dismissed due to time constraints.

Assessment Techniques

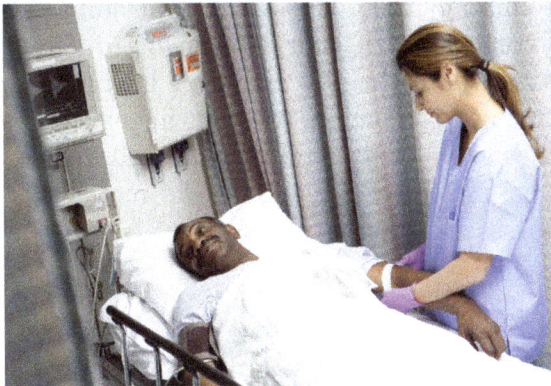

Inspection

Whether you are performing a comprehensive assessment or a focused assessment, you will use at least one of the following four basic techniques during your physical exam: inspection, auscultation, percussion, and palpation. These techniques should be used in an organized manner from least disturbing or invasive to most invasive to the patient.

Inspection is the most frequently used assessment technique. When you are using inspection, you are looking for conditions you can observe with your eyes, ears, or nose. Examples of things you may inspect are skin color, location of lesions, bruises or rash, symmetry, size of body parts and abnormal findings, sounds, and odors. Inspection can be an important technique as it leads to further investigation of findings.

Auscultation

Auscultation is usually performed following inspection, especially with abdominal assessment. The abdomen should be auscultated before percussion or palpation to prevent production of false bowel sounds.

When auscultating, ensure the exam room is quiet and auscultate over bare skin, listening to one sound at a time. Auscultation should never be performed over patient clothing or a gown, as it can produce false sounds or diminish true sounds. The bell or diaphragm of your stethoscope should be placed on your patient's skin firmly enough to leave a slight ring on the skin when removed.

Be aware that your patient's hair may also interfere with true identification of certain sounds. Remember to clean your stethoscope between patients.

The diaphragm is used to listen to high pitched sounds and the bell is best used to identify low pitched sounds.

Palpation

Palpation is another commonly used physical exam technique, requires you to touch your patient with different parts of your hand using different strength pressures. During light palpation, you press the skin about 1/2 inch to 3/4 inch with the pads of your fingers. When using deep palpation, use your finger pads and compress the skin approximately 1½ inches to 2 inches. Light palpation allows you to assess for texture, tenderness, temperature, moisture, pulsations, and masses. Deep palpation is performed to assess for masses and internal organs.

Percussion

Percussion is used to elicit tenderness or sounds that may provide clues to underlying problems.

When percussing directly over suspected areas of tenderness, monitor the patient for signs of discomfort. Percussion requires skill and practice.

The method of percussion is described as follows: Press the distal part of the middle finger of your non-dominant hand firmly on the body part. Keep the rest of your hand off the body surface. Flex the wrist, but not the foreman, of your dominant hand. Using the middle finger of your dominant hand, tap quickly and directly over the point where your other middle finger contacts the patient's skin, keeping the fingers perpendicular. Listen to the sounds produced.

These sounds may include:

- Tympany
- Resonance
- Hyperressonance
- Dullness
- Flatness

Tympany sounds like a drum and is heard over air pockets.

Resonance is a hollow sound heard over areas where there is a solid structure and some air (like the lungs).

Hyperressonance is a booming sound heard over air such as in emphysema. Dullness is heard over solid organs or masses.

Flatness is heard over dense tissues including muscle and bone.

Health History

The purpose of obtaining a health history is to provide you with a description of your patient's symptoms and how they developed. A complete history will serve as a guide to help identify potential or underlying illnesses or disease states. In addition to obtaining data about the patient's physical status, you will obtain information about many other factors that impact your patient's physical status including spiritual needs, cultural idiosyncrasies, and functional living status. The basic components of the complete health history (other than biographical information) include:

- Chief complaint
- Present health status
- Past health history
- Current lifestyle
- Psychosocial status
- Family history
- Review of systems.

Communication during the history and physical must be respectful and performed in a culturally-sensitive manner. Privacy is vital, and the healthcare professional needs to be aware of posture, body language, and tone of voice while interviewing the patient.

Chief Complaint

In your patient's own words, document the chief complaint. The chief complaint may be elicited by asking one of the following questions:

- So, tell me why you have come here today?

- Tell me what your biggest complaint is right now?

- What is bothering you the most right now?

- If we could fix any of your health problems right now, what would it be?

- What is giving you the most problems right now?

If your patient has more than one complaint, discuss which one is the most troublesome for them and document the complaints in order of importance as determined by the patient.

Present Health Status

Obtaining information about a patient's present health status allows the nurse to investigate current complaints. The mnemonic, PQRST, utilizes a structured format for information gathering, including evaluation of pain, and provides an efficient methodology to communicate with other healthcare providers. Use PQRST to assess each symptom and after any intervention to evaluate any changes or responses to treatment:

- Provocative or Palliative: What makes the symptom(s) better or worse?

- Quality: Describe the symptom(s).

- Region or Radiation: Where in the body does the symptom occur? Is there radiation or extension of the symptom(s) to another area of the body?

- Severity: On a scale of 1-10, (10 being the worst) how bad is the symptom(s)? Another visual scale may be appropriate for patients that are unable to identify with this scale.

- Timing: Does it occur in association with something else (i.e. eating, exertion, movement)?

Past Health History

It is important to ask questions about your patient's past health history. The past health history should elicit information about the patient's childhood illnesses and immunizations, accidents or traumatic injuries, hospitalizations, surgeries, psychiatric or mental illnesses, allergies, and chronic illnesses. For women, include history of menstrual cycle, how many pregnancies and how many births.

Childhood Illnesses: Data related to childhood illnesses is more pertinent to children than adults and the elderly. For adults, you want to know if they have ever had rheumatic fever and if their tetanus and hepatitis B vaccinations are current. For the elderly, you may want to ask if they ever had polio, rheumatic fever, or chicken pox. Pertinent vaccinations for the elderly would include tetanus, pneumonia and influenza.

Accidents or Traumatic Injuries: When assessing this area of the past health history, pay particular attention to patterns of injury, especially in infants, children, women and the elderly.

Hospitalizations: Be sure to ask the reason for the hospitalization and the nature of the treatments received while in the hospital such as blood transfusions, surgeries and any follow-up treatments. Remember to include hospitalizations for childbirth.

Surgeries: Many surgical procedures are performed on an outpatient basis. Questions regarding surgeries should also be asked in addition to hospitalizations, as patients may not discuss a surgery if there was no associated hospital stay.

Psychiatric or Mental Illnesses: If your patient has a past history of psychiatric or mental illnesses, ask what triggered the illness, if anything, and the course and the progression of the illness. This includes depression and anxiety, as well as diagnosed mental illness.

Allergies: Identify what your patient is allergic to (both food and medication), as well as the reaction and response to treatment. It is important to ask about any environmental allergies or sensitivities (such as latex).

Family History

Family history is important in identifying your patient's risk for certain disease states.

Applicable generations with whom to explore health status include grandparents, parents, and the children of your patient.

Chronic illnesses or known diseases with genetic components should also be screened for. Chronic illness or disease can include cancer, diabetes, autoimmune disorders, cholesterol, heart disease, hypertension, renal disease, and mental illness, among others.

Current Health Status

Information collected should also include details about your patient's personal habits such as smoking or drinking, nutrition, cholesterol, and if there is a history of heart disease or hypertension.

Medications

Obtain a list of current medications, including dose and frequency, as well as reason for taking them. Remember to ask the patient about over the counter medications, vitamins, and herbal supplements.

Review of Systems and Physical Exam

The physical examination can be performed in a "head-to-toe" fashion, starting with the head and ending with the toes. Although some healthcare professionals have varied tactics to performing this skill, the key to assessment is to ensure a consistent, methodical approach to avoid missing any vital assessment areas.

A physical examination should include:

- Complete set of vital signs (blood pressure, heart rate, respiratory rate and temperature)

- Assess immediate pain level. Can use acronym "PQRST" for quick pain assessment:

    o P=provoking factors (what brought on the pain?)

    o Q=quality (describe the pain- i.e. stabbing, throbbing, burning)

    o R=radiation (does the pain radiate anywhere?)

    o S=severity/symptoms (how bad is the pain-rate it; are there other symptoms with the pain?)

    o T=timing (is it constant? What makes it better/worse?)

A review of systems can be incorporated during your physical exam. While examining each body system, it is appropriate to ask certain history questions that pertain to that system. The areas in parentheses are clues or details to note in each area.

Skin Assessment

Skin assessment can be performed throughout the physical examination. As each body system is examined, assessment of the skin can be incorporated into findings.

When assessing the skin, examine the following:

- General pigmentation (evenness, appropriate for heritage)

- Systemic color changes (pallor, erythema, cyanosis, jaundice)

- Freckles and moles (symmetry, size, border, pigmentation)

- Temperature (hypothermia, hyperthermia)

- Moisture and texture (diaphoresis, dehydration, firm smooth texture)

- Edema (location and degree)

- Bruising (location, pattern, consistent with history – especially in at risk populations)

- Lesions (color, elevation, pattern or shape, size, location, exudates)

- Hair (normal color, texture, distribution)

- Nails (shape, contour, color)

- Remember that skin breakdown is a common problem with ill and hospitalized patients. Skin assessment is vital to identify areas of vulnerability in the prevention of pressure ulcer.

Neurological Assessment

It may not be necessary to perform the entire neurological exam on a patient with no suspicion of neurological disorders. You should perform a complete baseline neurological examination on any patient that has verbalized neurological concerns in their history, or if a noted neurological deficit is discovered. When examining the nervous system, ask the following:

- Any past history of head injury? (location, loss of consciousness)

- Do you have frequent or severe headaches? (when, where, how often)

- Any dizziness or vertigo? (frequency, precipitating factors, gradual or sudden)

- Ever had/or do you have seizures? (when did they start, frequency, course and duration, motor activity associated with, associated signs, postictal phase, precipitating factors, medications, coping strategies)

- Any difficulty swallowing? (solids or liquids, excessive saliva)

- Any difficulty speaking? (forming words or actually saying what you intended)

- Do you have any coordination problems? (describe)

- Do you have any numbness or tingling? (describe)

- Any significant past neurologic history? (cerebral vascular accident, spinal cord injuries, neurologic infections, congenital disorders)

- Environmental or occupational hazards? (insecticides, lead, organic solvents, illicit drugs, alcohol).

Recheck the neurological exam at periodic intervals with any patient that has a neurological deficit.

The Complete Neurological Exam

When performing the complete neurological exam, examine the following 12 cranial nerves:

- Cranial Nerve I: Olfactory

- Cranial Nerve II: Optic

- Cranial Nerves III, IV, & VI: Oculomotor

- Trochlear, and Abducens

- Cranial Nerve V: Trigeminal

- Cranial Nerve VII: Facial Nerve

- Cranial Nerve VIII: Acoustic (Vestibulocochlear)

- Cranial Nerve IX & X: Glossopharyngeal and Vagus

- Cranial Nerve XI: Spinal Accessory

- Cranial Nerve XII: Hypoglossal.

Inspect and palpate the motor system

(Tests muscle groups and for motor neuron disease)

- Muscles appropriate size for body (atrophy, hypertrophy)

- Muscle strength (asymmetric, weak for patient)

- Muscle tone (range of motion, pain, flaccidity, spasticity, rigidity)

- Involuntary movements (tic, tremor, fasciculation).

Check Cerebellar Function

(Tests balance and coordination and skilled movements)

- Gait (stiff posture, staggering, wide base of support, lack of arm swing, unequal steps, dragging or slapping of foot, ataxia)

- Romberg's test (loss of balance increases when eyes are closed)

- Rapid alternating movements (lack of coordination, slow, clumsy)

- Finger to finger test (misses mark)

- Finger to nose test (misses mark)

- Heel to shin test (misses mark, lower extremity coordination impaired).

Assess the Sensory System

(Tests intactness of peripheral nerves, sensory tracts, and higher cortical discrimination)

- Superficial pain

- Light touch

- Vibration.

Assess the Spinothalmic Tract

(Tests for ability to sense pain, temperature, and light touch)

- Presence of pain (hypoalgesia, hyperalgesia, analgesia)

- Temperature (test only if pain test is normal)

- Light touch (hypoesthesia, anesthesia, hyperesthesia).

Assess Posterior Column Tract

(May identify lesions of the sensory cortex or vertebral column)

- Vibration

- Position

- Tactile discrimination (stereognosis, graphesthesia)

- Two point discrimination.

Check the Reflexes

(May identify upper motor neuron disease, diseases of the pyramidal tract, or spinal cord injury)

- Stretch or deep tendon reflexes (clonus, hyporeflexia, hyperreflexia)

- Superficial reflexes (Abdominal, cremasteric, plantar).

The Neurological Recheck or Abbreviated Neurological Exam

Perform the neurological recheck exam at periodic intervals with your patient that has a neurologic deficit. This exam is also useful for your inpatient with a head injury or systemic disease process that may be manifesting as a neurologic symptom.

When performing this abbreviated exam, examine the following which are mentioned below.

Level of Consciousness

(Monitors for signs of increasing intracranial pressure)

- Is your patient oriented to person, place, and time? Are they oriented to the situation?

- Is your patient alert? If not, what does it take to get them alert - calling their name, light touch, vigorous touch, pain?

Motor Function

- Ask your patient to squeeze your fingers with their hands and let go (tests for strength and symmetry of strength in the upper extremities).

- Ask your patient to push and pull their arms toward and away from you when their elbows are bent. Provide some resistance (tests for strength and symmetry of strength in upper extremities).

- Ask your patient to dorsiflex and plantarflex their feet, while providing some resistance (tests for strength and symmetry of strength in lower extremities).

- Ask your patient to perform straight leg raises with and without resistance (tests for strength and symmetry of strength in lower extremities).

Pupillary Response

- Size, shape, and symmetry of both pupils should be the same.

- Each pupil should constrict briskly when a light is shined into the eyes.

- Each pupil should have consensual light reflex.

Glasgow Coma Scale

The Glasgow Coma Scale assesses how the brain functions as a whole and not as individual parts.

The scale assesses three major brain functions:

- Eye opening

- Motor response

- Verbal response.

A completely normal person will score 15 on the scale overall. Scores of less than 7 reflect coma. Using the scale consistently in the healthcare setting allows healthcare providers to share a common language and monitor for trends across time.

Glasgow Coma Scale (GCS)	
Best Eye Opening Response	1 = No response
	2 = To pain
	3 = To speech
	4 = Spontaneously
Best Motor Response	1 = No response
	2 = Extension – abnormal
	3 = Flexion - abnormal
	4 = Flexion – withdrawal
	5 = Localizes pain
	6 = Obeys verbal commands
Best Verbal Response	1 = No response
	2 = Sounds -
	3 = Speech - inappropriate
	4 = Conversation - confused
	5 = Oriented X 3

Head, Face and Throat Assessment

When assessing the head, face and throat, focus on assessment of suspected deficits as indicated by the history, patient complaints, or disease process the patient is exhibiting. Some of the following points fall outside of the general scope of nursing practice but may be observed by the nurse, or practiced in advanced nursing roles. A complete exam of the head, face and throat is not warranted in every patient.

When examining the head, ears, eyes, nose, mouth, and throat, ask the following questions:

- Do you get frequent or severe headaches?

- Any past history of head injury?

- Do you frequently get dizzy?

- Do you have any neck pain, swelling, or lumps?

- Do you have a history of head or neck

- Surgery?

Look for:

- General facial symmetry
- Hair distribution
- General facial expressions
- Lymph nodes or lesions.

Assessment of the Eyes

Eyes

- Any vision changes or difficulty?
- Any eye pain?
- Do you have double vision?
- Any redness, swelling or discharge?
- Do you have a history of glaucoma?
- Do you wear glasses or contacts?

Look for:

- Visual acuity
- Visual fields (confrontation test)
- Extraocular muscle function (nystagmus, abnormal corneal light reflex)
- Conjunctiva and sclera (redness, irritation)
- Pupil (shape, symmetry, light reflexes, accommodation)
- Ocular fundus (red reflex, optic disc, retinal vessels, macula).

Assessment of the Ears

Ears

- Have you had many ear infections?
- Do you have any discharge from your ears?
- Do you have any hearing difficulty?
- Do you have any environmental or occupational exposure to loud noises?
- Any ringing in your ears (tinnitus)?
- Any dizziness (vertigo)?

Look for:

- Size, shape, skin condition, and tenderness
- External canal (redness, swelling, discharge)
- Tympanic membrane [color & characteristics (amber, redness), air/fluid levels]
- Hearing acuity (also examined as you collect the patient's history).

Assessment of the Nose

Nose

- Any nasal discharge?
- Do you get frequent colds?
- Do you have sinus pain?
- Do you get nose bleeds?
- Do you have allergies?
- Have you had a change in sense of smell?

Look for:

- Nasal cavity (discharge, rhinnorhea, swollen, boggy, mucosa)
- Sinuses (tenderness and transillumination).

Assessment of the Mouth and Throat

Mouth and Throat

- Skin integrity (lesions or blisters)
- Teeth (discoloration, bleeding or swollen gums)
- Tongue (color, surface characteristics, moisture, lesions)
- Buccal mucosa (discoloration, Koplik's spots, leukoplakia)
- Uvula (midline)
- Throat (tonsils, Cranial Nerve XII by sticking out tongue).

Look For:

- Do you have any sores or lesions in your mouth or throat?
- Do you have a sore throat and hoarseness?

- Do you have a toothache or get bleeding gums?

- Any difficulty swallowing?

- Do things taste differently than usual?

- Do you smoke, drink or chew tobacco?

Cardiovascular Assessment

Cardiovascular disease is the United States' leading killer for both men and women among all racial and ethnic groups. In 2009, heart disease is estimated to cost more than $304.6 billion, including health care services, medications, and lost productivity. Therefore, a complete cardiovascular exam should be a part of every abbreviated and complete assessment.

When examining the cardiovascular system, ask about the following:

- Any chest pain? (use PQRST pneumonic)

- Do you ever get short of breath? (associated with what)

- How many pillows do you sleep on at night? (orthopnea)

- Do you have a cough? (describe, frequency, timing, severity, sputum production)

- Are you frequently fatigued? (morning or night)

- Do you have any swelling or skin color changes? (edema, cyanosis, pallor)

- How often do you get up at night to urinate? (nocturia)

- Do you have a past history of cardiac or cardiovascular events or disorders?

- Do you have a family history of cardiovascular disease?

- Assess cardiac risk factors?

When assessing the cardiovascular system, examine the following:

- Palpate and auscultate the carotid artery (strength of pulsation, bruits, murmurs).

- Inspect and palpate the jugular veins (jugular vein distention).

- Inspect the precordium (heaves, lifts).

- Palpate the precordium (location of apical impulse, presence of thrill).

- Percuss cardiac borders.

- Auscultate heart sounds.

  ○ Auscultate in a Z-pattern listening over the aortic, pulmonic, mitral, and tricuspid valves and over Erb's point)

  ○ Identify S1 and S2.

  ○ Listen to S1 and S2 separately (split S1 or S2).

  ○ Listen for any extra heart sounds (S3, S4, clicks, rubs).

  ○ Listen for murmurs (note timing/loudness/pitch/pattern/quality/location/radiation/position).

- Palpate peripheral pulses: brachial, radial, femoral, popliteal, dorsalis pedis, posterior tibial (strength and symmetry).

- Inspect extremities (color, capillary refill, edema, ulcerations).

Pulmonary Assessment

When examining the pulmonary system, ask the following for both abbreviated and complete examinations:

- Do you have a cough? (use PQRST pneumonic)

- Do you frequently get short of breath? (position, associated night sweats, related to any triggering event)

- Pain with breathing? (constant or periodic, describe the quality, treatment)

- Any past history of breathing trouble or lung disease? (frequency and severity of colds, allergies, asthma family history, smoking, environmental or occupational risk factors).

When examining the pulmonary system, explore the following as indicated by your patient's history, symptoms or disease processes they are exhibiting:

- Inspect the thoracic cage (symmetry of expansion, anterior-posterior diameter, any areas of retractions)

- Palpate the thoracic cage (tactile fremitus)

- Percuss the thoracic cage (hyperressonance, dullness, diaphragmatic excursion)

- Auscultate the anterior and posterior chest:

  ○ Have patient breath slightly deeper than normal through their mouth

- ○ Auscultate from C-7 to approximately T-8, in a left to right comparative sequence. You should auscultate between every rib.

- ○ Listen for bronchial, bronchovesicular, and vesicular breath sounds

- ○ Identify any adventitious breath sounds, their location, and timing in relation to the cardiac cycle (crackles, or rales and wheezes or rhonchi)

- Auscultate voice sounds including bronchophony, egophony and whispered pectoriloquy

Assessing the Abdomen/Gastrointestinal System

When examining the abdomen/gastrointestinal system, ASK about the following:

- Any change in appetite?

- Any difficulty swallowing? (dysphagia)

- Any abdominal pain? (use PQRST pneumonic)

- Any nausea or vomiting? (color, odor, presence of blood, food intake in past 24 hours)

- Any change in bowel habits? (constipation, diarrhea, blood in stool, or dark, tarry stools)

- Do you have any hemorrhoids? (bleeding, treatment)

- Any past history of abdominal problems? (gall bladder, liver, pancreas, digestion, elimination)

When assessing the abdomen, examine the following:

- Inspect for bulges, masses, hernias, ascites, spider nevi, veins, pulsations or movements, inability to lie flat.

- Auscultate after inspection so you do not produce false bowel sound through percussion or palpation. Auscultate for bowel sounds (normal, hyper- or hypo-active) and bruits.

- Percuss for general tympany, liver span, splenic dullness (dullness over the spleen), costovertebral angle tenderness, presence of fluid wave and shifting dullness with ascites.

- Palpate lightly then deeply noting any muscle guarding, rigidity, masses or tenderness. Palpate tender areas last.

- Palpate the liver margins (often it is not palpable).

- Palpate the spleen (enlargement occurs with mononucleosis and trauma).

- Palpate the kidneys (enlargement may indicate a mass).

- Assess for rebound tenderness (pain on release of pressure to the abdomen usually indicates peritoneal irritation).

- When acute abdominal pain is present perform the iliopsoas muscle test and obturator test.

Musculoskeletal System

When examining the musculoskeletal system, ask the following:

- Any joint pain or problems? (Use PQRST pneumonic.)

- Any stiffness in your joints? Any swelling, heat or redness in your joints?

- Any limitation of movement in your joints?

- Which activities are difficult? (Assess functional ability.)

- Any muscle problems (pain, cramping, aches, weakness, atrophy)?

- Any bone problems (bone pain, deformity, history of broken bones)?

When assessing the musculoskeletal system,examine the following:

- Inspect the size and shape of any problem joints (color, swelling, masses,deformities).

- Palpate each joint for temperature and range of motion (heat, tenderness,swelling, masses, limitation in range of motion, crepitation).

- Test muscle strength and strength against resistance of the major muscle groups of the body. Assess the temporomandibular joint (swelling, crepitus, pain).

- Assess the cervical spine (alignment of head and neck, symmetry of muscles, tenderness, spasms, range of motion).

- Inspect and assess upper extremity strength and range of motion for the shoulders, elbows, wrists, and hands.

- Inspect and assess lower extremity strength and range of motion for the hips, knees, ankles and feet.

Male Reproductive System

When examining the reproductive systems, ask about the following:

- Do you urinate more than usual? (frequency, urgency, nocturia)

- Any pain or burning upon urination?

- Any difficulty starting or maintaining the stream of urine?

- Any difficulty controlling you urine? Any blood in your urine?

- Any problems with you penis? (pain, lesions, discharge)

- Any problems with your scrotum? (lumps, tenderness, swelling)

- Are you in a sexually active relationship and if so any difficulties in this relationship related to the physical act of intercourse?

- Do you use contraceptives? (what type, questions or concerns)

- Any sexual contact with a partner whom may have had a sexually transmitted disease?

- Do you perform self-testicular examinations monthly?

When assessing the male reproductive system, examine the following:

- Inspect and palpate the penis (inflammation, lesions, freely moveable foreskin in uncircumcised male, location of urinary meatus, pubic lice or nits, narrowed urethral opening).

- Inspect and palpate the scrotum (scrotal edema, lesions or inflammation, absent, atrophied or fixed testes, tenderness of testicle or spermatic cord).

- Inspect and palpate for hernia.

- Inspect and palpate inguinal lymph nodes.

- Discuss and encourage self-testicular exams monthly.

Female Reproductive System

When examining the reproductive systems, ask about the following:

- Do you urinate more than usual? (frequency, urgency, nocturia); Any pain or burning upon urination?

- Any difficulty starting or maintaining the stream of urine?

- Any blood in your urine? Any difficulty controlling you urine?

- Any unusual vaginal discharge?

- Are you sexually active? Any difficulties related to the physical act of intercourse?

- Do you use contraceptives? (what type, questions or concerns)

- Any sexual contact with a partner whom may have had a sexually transmitted disease?

- Tell me about your menstrual history (onset, length, amount of flow, cramps, bloating, PMS, age of first period, age of menopause).

- Have you ever been pregnant? (if so how many times, how many live births, any miscarriages or abortions, any complications)

- Have your periods slowed down or stopped? (associated symptoms of menopause, estrogen replacement therapy, psychological well-being)

- Any breast tenderness, lumps, discharge or concerns? Do you perform self-breast examinations monthly?

- Do you have regular PAP smears?

The complete female reproductive system examination is usually only performed by specially trained nurses or a physician. Please consider the following when examining the female reproductive system:

In the lithotomy position examine the external genitalia:

- Skin color

- Hair distribution

- Labia and clitoris (swelling, lesions)

- Urethral opening (stricture, inflammation)

- Vaginal opening (foul-smelling discharge, inflammation, lesions)

- Palpate the vagina (tenderness, swelling, discharge, Bartholin's glands).

The internal genitalia are only examined by specially trained healthcare providers, but you may be requested to assist with a vaginal examination. This would include assisting with the speculum to visualize the cervix (color, position, size, cervical os, surface of cervix, cervical secretions), and obtaining cervical smears and cultures. A bimanual (rectal - vaginal) exam may be performed to rule out rectal disease.

Cervix should be smooth, firm, round, and mobile. Uterus and adnexa should not be enlarged, tender, fixed, or nodular. Ovaries are often not palpable, but if they are, they should be small, round and smooth. Your patient may feel a slight pang or twinge upon palpation and should resolve quickly.

Examine the breasts and axilla:

- Inspect the breasts for size, symmetry, and nipple dimpling.

- Palpate the breasts and axilla in a circular pattern, covering all areas (note inconsistencies and tenderness).

- If you palpate a mass, note its size, shape, consistency, mobility, degree of tenderness, and location.

Nutritional Assessment

Assessing nutritional status of your patients is important for several reasons. A thorough nutritional assessment will identify individuals at risk for malnutrition and provide baseline information for nutritional assessments in the future. A nutritional screening is indicated for all patients. A complete nutritional assessment is indicated for only those individuals at risk for malnutrition. A screening assessment includes:

- Biographical Data

  - Age

  - Height

  - Weight

- Lab Data

  - Albumin

  - Hemoglobin

  - Hematocrit

  - Total lymphocytes

  - Other abnormal labs?

Signs of Malnutrition

When performing your physical exam, observe for the following signs and symptoms of nutritional deficiency:

- Eyes dry

- Pale or red conjunctivae

- Blepharitis

- Cheilosis

- Cracks at the side of mouth

- Tongue pale

- Bleeding gums

- Dry, flaky skin

- Petichiae

- Bruising

- Dry, bumpy skin

- Petechiae

- Cracked skin

- Eczema

- Xanthomas

- Dull, dry, thin hair

- Hair color changes

- Brittle nails

- Joint pain

- Muscle wasting

- Pain in calves

- Splinter hemorrhages of nails

- Peripheral neuropathy

- Hyporeflexia

- Confusion or irritability.

Putting it All Together

Once nurses are familiar with the health assessment of the adult, it is necessary to adapt the assessment for specific patients such as infants, children, and the elderly. Knowledge of Age-specific considerations will allow the nurse to evaluate the significance of the health history and exam results and apply specifics to an individualized plan of care.

References

- Potter, Patricia A.; Perry, Anne Griffin; Stockert, Patricia A.; Hall, Amy M. (2013). Fundamentals of Nursing (8 ed.). St. Louis: Mosby. p. 222. ISBN 978-0-323-07933-4.

- Health-assessment, file-manager: nchk.org.hk, Retrieved 28 May 2018

- Zarzycka, D; Górajek-Jóźwik, J (2004). "Nursing diagnosis with the ICNP in the teaching context". International Nursing Review. 51 (4): 240–49. doi:10.1111/j.1466-7657.2004.00249.x. PMID 15530164.

- Weir-Hughes, Dickon (2010). "Nursing Diagnosis in Administration". Nursing Diagnoses 2009–2011, Custom: Definitions and Classification. John Wiley & Sons. pp. 37–40. ISBN 978-1-4443-2727-4.

- Glossary-of-Terms: kb.nanda.org, Retrieved 16 June 2018

- Lunney, Margaret (2008). "The Need for International Nursing Diagnosis Research and a Theoretical Framework". International Journal of Nursing Terminologies and Classifications. 19 (1): 28–34. doi:10.1111/j.1744-618X.2007.00076.x. PMID 18331482.

Vital Assessment

An examination and measurement of a patient's vital signs such as body temperature, pulse, blood pressure and respiratory rate is called a vital assessment. It is an important area of nursing assessment. This chapter discusses all aspects of vital assessment performed by a nurse through an analysis of the major vital signs and their assessment techniques.

Vital Signs

Vital signs are measurements of the body's most basic functions. The four main vital signs routinely monitored by medical professionals and health care providers include the following:

- Body temperature
- Pulse rate
- Respiration rate (rate of breathing)
- Blood pressure (Blood pressure is not considered a vital sign, but is often measured along with the vital signs.)

Vital signs are useful in detecting or monitoring medical problems. Vital signs can be measured in a medical setting, at home, at the site of a medical emergency, or elsewhere.

Body Temperature

The normal body temperature of a person varies depending on gender, recent activity, food and fluid consumption, time of day, and, in women, the stage of the menstrual cycle. Normal body temperature can range from 97.8° F (36.5° C) to 99° F (37.2° C) for a healthy adult. A person's body temperature can be taken in any of the following ways:

- Orally: Temperature can be taken by mouth using either the classic glass thermometer, or the more modern digital thermometers that use an electronic probe to measure body temperature.

- Rectally: Temperatures taken rectally (using a glass or digital thermometer) tend to be 0.5° F to 0.7° F higher than when taken by mouth.

- Armpit (axillary): Temperatures can be taken under the arm using a glass or digital thermometer. Temperatures taken by this route tend to be 0.3° F to 0.4° F lower than those temperatures taken by mouth.

- By ear: A special thermometer can quickly measure the temperature of the eardrum, which reflects the body's core temperature (the temperature of the internal organs).

- By skin: A special thermometer can quickly measure the temperature of the skin on the forehead.

Body temperature may be abnormal due to fever (high temperature) or hypothermia (low temperature). A fever is indicated when body temperature rises about one degree or more over the normal temperature of 98.6° F, according to the American Academy of Family Physicians. Hypothermia is defined as a drop in body temperature below 95° F.

Pulse

This can be measured at any place where there is a large artery (e.g. carotid, femoral, or simply by listening over the heart), though for the sake of convenience it is generally done by palpating the radial impulse. You may find it helpful to feel both radial arteries simultaneously, doubling the sensory input and helping to insure the accuracy of your measurements. Place the tips of your index and middle fingers just proximal to the patients wrist on the thumb side, orienting them so that they are both over the length of the vessel.

Vascular Anatomy

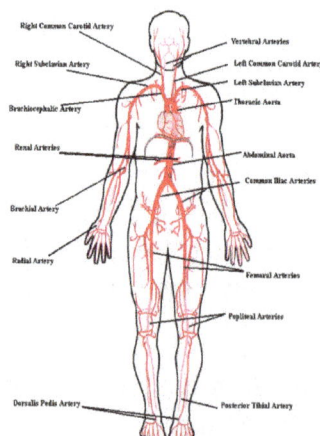

Technique for Measuring the Radial Pulse

The pictures below demonstrate the location of the radial artery (surface anatomy on the left, gross anatomy on the right).

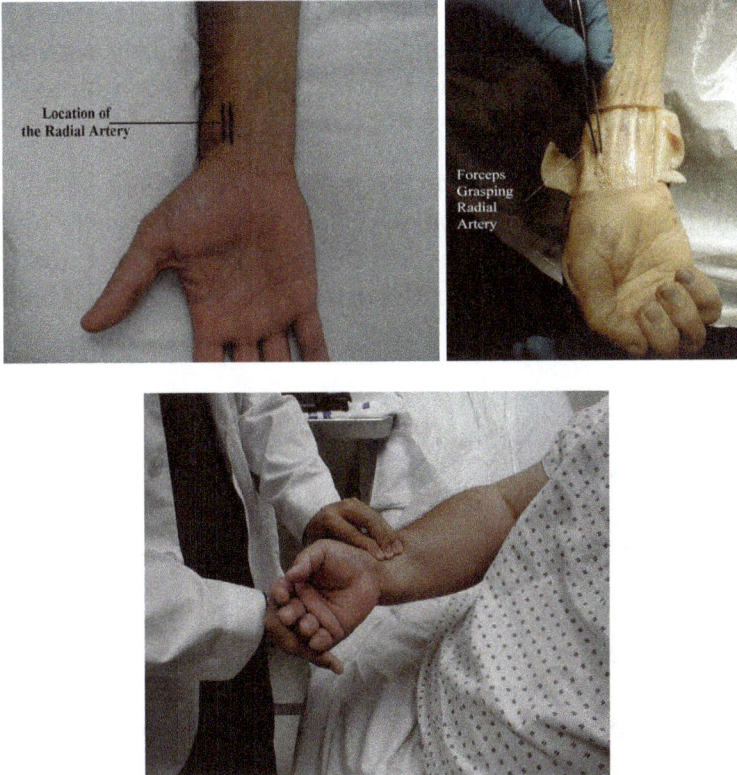

Location of the Radial Artery

Forceps Grasping Radial Artery

Frequently, you can see transmitted pulsations on careful visual inspection of this region, which may help in locating this artery. Upper extremity peripheral vascular disease is relatively uncommon, so the radial artery should be readily palpable in most patients. Push lightly at first, adding pressure if there is a lot of subcutaneous fat or you are unable to detect a pulse. If you push too hard, you might occlude the vessel and mistake your own pulse for that of the patient. During palpation, note the following:

1. Quantity: Measure the rate of the pulse (recorded in beats per minute). Count for 30 seconds and multiply by 2 (or 15 seconds x 4). If the rate is particularly slow or fast, it is probably best to measure for a full 60 seconds in order to minimize the impact of any error in recording over shorter periods of time. Normal is between 60 and 100.

2. Regularity: Is the time between beats constant? In the normal setting, the heart rate should appear metronomic. Irregular rhythms, however, are quite common. If the pattern is entirely chaotic with no discernable pattern, it is referred to as irregularly irregular and likely represents atrial fibrillation.

Extra beats can also be added into the normal pattern, in which case the rhythm is described as regularly irregular. This may occur, for example, when impulses originating from the ventricle are interposed at regular junctures on the normal rhythm. If the pulse is irregular, it's a good idea to verify the rate by listening over the heart. This is because certain rhythm disturbances do not allow adequate ventricular filling with each beat. The resultant systole may generate a rather small stroke volume whose impulse is not palpable in the periphery.

3. Volume: Does the pulse volume (i.e. the subjective sense of fullness) feel normal? This reflects changes in stroke volume. In the setting of hypovolemia, for example, the pulse volume is relatively low (aka weak or thready). There may even be beat to beat variation in the volume, occurring occasionally with systolic heart failure.

Respiratory Rate

Respiratory rate should be taken for *one full minute*. Auscultation with a stethoscope will increase the ability to hear shallow breaths.

Respiratory rhythm and depth should be evaluated using a manual assessment and observation of the patient's respiratory pattern. Visualization of the chest wall effectively enables the evaluation of accessory muscle use. Respiratory effort is described in the table below.

Normal	Normal effort no in-drawing, no apnea
Mild	Mild increased respiratory effort, nasal flaring, mild-in-drawing
Moderate	Moderately increased rep. effort, nasal flaring, marked in-drawing with multiple muscle groups
Severe	Greatly increased respiratory effort, in-drawing, audible grunt, nasal flaring, head bobbing,tracheal tug, accessory muscle use, apneas

Blood Pressure

Blood pressure is the force of the blood pushing against the artery walls during contraction and relaxation of the heart. Each time the heart beats, it pumps blood into the arteries, resulting in the highest blood pressure as the heart contracts. When the heart relaxes, the blood pressure falls.

Two numbers are recorded when measuring blood pressure. The higher number, or systolic pressure, refers to the pressure inside the artery when the heart contracts and pumps blood through the body. The lower number, or diastolic pressure, refers to the pressure inside the artery when the heart is at rest and is filling with blood. Both the systolic and diastolic pressures are recorded as "mm Hg" (millimeters of mercury). This recording represents how high the mercury column in an old-fashioned manual blood pressure device (called a mercury manometer or sphygmomanometer) is raised by the pressure of the blood. Today, your nurse's office is more likely to use a simple dial for this measurement.

High blood pressure, or hypertension, directly increases the risk of heart attack, heart failure, and stroke. With high blood pressure, the arteries may have an increased resistance against the flow of blood, causing the heart to pump harder to circulate the blood.

Blood pressure is categorized as normal, elevated, or stage 1 or stage 2 high blood pressure:

- Normal blood pressure is systolic of less than 120 and diastolic of less than 80 (120/80)

- Elevated blood pressure is systolic of 120 to 129 and diastolic less than 80

- Stage 1 high blood pressure is systolic is 130 to 139 or diastolic between 80 to 89

- Stage 2 high blood pressure is when systolic is 140 or higher or the diastolic is 90 or higher.

These numbers should be used as a guide only. A single blood pressure measurement that is higher than normal is not necessarily an indication of a problem. Your nurse will want to see multiple blood pressure measurements over several days or weeks before making a diagnosis of high blood pressure and starting treatment. Ask your provider when to contact him or her if your blood pressure readings are not within normal range.

Fifth Vital Signs

The "fifth vital sign" may refer to a few different parameters.:

- Pain is considered a standard fifth vital sign in some organizations such as the U.S. Veterans Affairs. Pain is measured on a pain scale based on subjective patient reporting and may be unreliable. Some studies show that recording pain routinely may not change management.

- Menstrual cycle

- Pulse Oximetry

- Blood Glucose level.

Sixth Vital Signs

There is no standard "sixth vital sign"; its use is more informal and discipline-dependent than the above:

- End-tidal CO_2

- Functional status

- Shortness of breath

- Gait speed.

Process of Assessing Vital Signs

Assessing Vital Signs

Steps

1. Temperature:

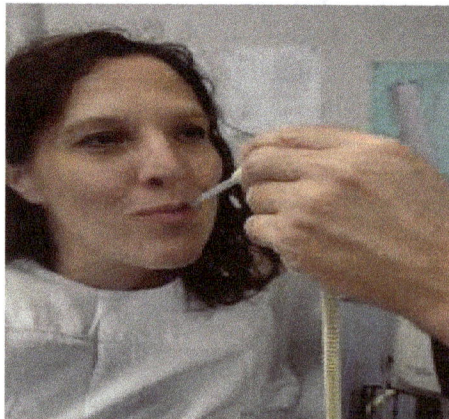

Normal (oral) = 35.8° C to 37.3° C.

Oral temperature: Place the thermometer in the mouth under the tongue and instruct patient to keep mouth closed. Leave the thermometer in place for as long as is indicated by the device manufacturer.

Axillary temperature: Usually 1° C lower than oral temperature. Place the thermometer in patient's armpit and leave it in place for as long as is indicated by the device manufacturer.

Tympanic membrane (ear) temperature: Usually 0.3° C to 0.6° C higher than an oral temperature. The tympanic membrane shares the same vascular artery that perfuses the hypothalamus. Do not force the thermometer into the ear and do not occlude the ear canal.

Rectal temperature: Usually 1° C higher than oral temperature. Use only when other routes are not available.

2. Pulse:

Normal resting heart rate = 60 to 100 beats per minute.

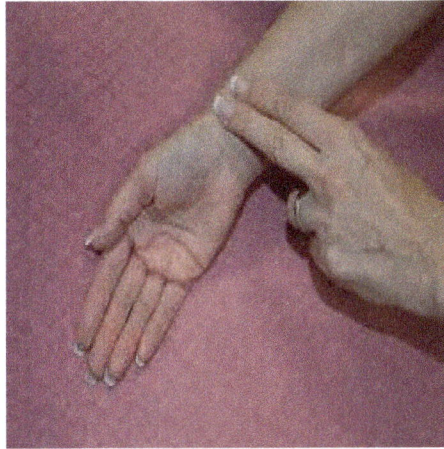

Radial pulse

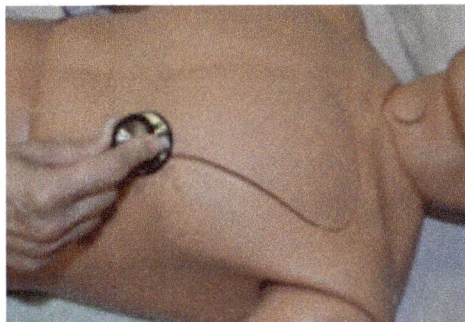

Apical pulse

Radial pulse: Use the pads of your first three fingers to gently palpate the radial pulse at the inner lateral wrist.

Apical pulse: Taken as part of a focused cardiovascular assessment and when the pulse rate is irregular. Apical heart rate should be used as the parameter indicated in certain cardiac medications (e.g., digoxin). Apical pulse rate should be taken for a full minute for accuracy, and is located at the fifth intercostal space in line with the middle of the clavicle in adults.

Carotid pulse: May be taken when radial pulse is not present or is difficult to palpate.

3. Respiration rate:

Normal resting respiratory rate = 10 to 20 breaths per minute.

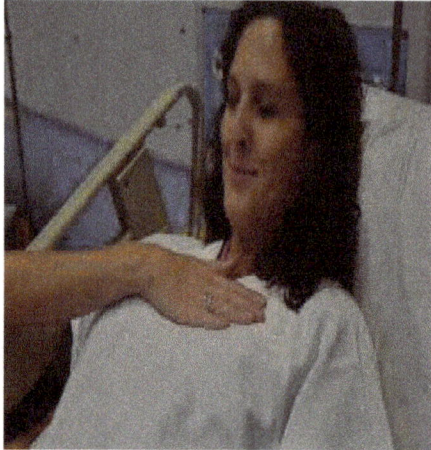

Count respiratory rate unobtrusively while you are taking the pulse rate so that the patient is not aware that you are taking the respiration rate. Count for 30 seconds or for a full minute if irregular.

4. Blood pressure (BP):

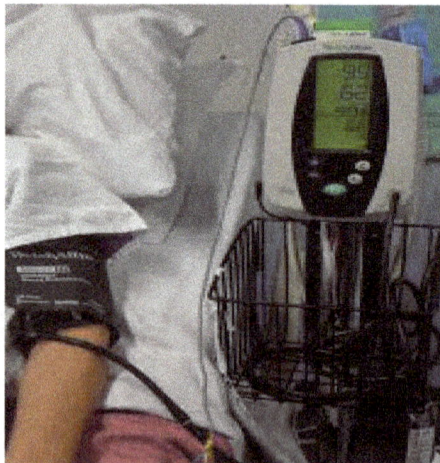

Blood pressure cuff

The average BP for an adult is 120/80 mmHg, but variations are normal for various reasons.

The systolic pressure is the maximum pressure on the arteries during left ventricular contraction.

The diastolic pressure is the resting pressure on the arteries between each cardiac contraction.

The patient may be sitting or lying down with the bare arm at heart level. Palpate the brachial artery just above the antecubital fossa medially. Wrap the BP cuff around the upper arm about 2.5 cm above the brachial artery.

Palpate the radial or brachial artery, and inflate the BP cuff until the pulse rate is no longer felt. Then inflate 20 to 30 mmHg more.

Place the bell of the stethoscope over the brachial artery, and deflate the cuff slowly and evenly, noting the points at which you hear the first appearance of sound (systolic BP), and the disappearance of sound (diastolic BP).

References

- National Early Warning Score Development and Implementation Group (NEWSDIG) (2012). National Early Warning Score (NEWS): standardising the assessment of acute-illness severity in the NHS. London: Royal College of Physicians. ISBN 978-1-86016-471-2

- Vital-signs-body-temperature-pulse-rate-respiration-rate-blood-pressure-85: hopkinsmedicine.org, Retrieved 09 July 2018

- Mower W, Sachs C, Nicklin E, Baraff L (1997). "Pulse oximetry as a fifth pediatric vital sign". Pediatrics. 99 (5): 681–6. doi:10.1542/peds.99.5.681. PMID 9113944

- Vitals, module-two-clinical-care, Nursing-Student-Orientation, Education-and-learning: sickkids.ca, Retrieved 29 March 2018

- "Mining Vital Signs from Wearable Healthcare Device via Nonlinear Machine Learning". University of Hull. Retrieved 2016-05-14

- Neff T (1988). "Routine oximetry. A fifth vital sign?". Chest. 94 (2): 227. doi:10.1378/chest.94.2.227a. PMID 3396392

- Vital-signs, clinical-skills: pentextbc.ca, Retrieved 18 May 2018

- "Nursing care of dyspnea: the 6th vital sign in individuals with chronic obstructive pulmonary disease (COPD)". National Guideline Clearinghouse. Archived from the original on 2009-01-17. Retrieved 2009-01-16

Physical Assessment

The medical investigation of a person's body in search of any signs or symptoms of a disease falls under physical examination. This chapter provides an overview of physical examination and the head-to-toe assessment of a patient that a nurse undertakes to gather crucial information regarding the patient's health.

Physical Examination

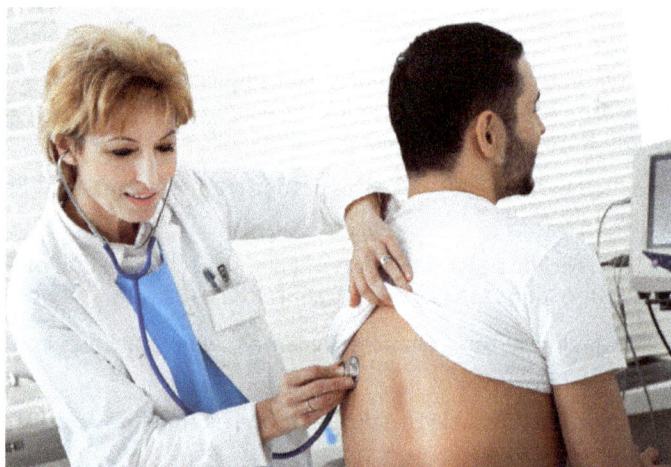

A physical examination is a routine test your primary care provider (PCP) performs to check your overall health. A PCP may be a doctor, a nurse practitioner, or a physician assistant. The exam is also known as a wellness check. You don't have to be sick to request an exam.

The physical exam can be a good time to ask your PCP questions about your health or discuss any changes or problems that you have noticed.

There are different tests that can be performed during your physical examination. Depending on your age or medical or family history, your PCP may recommend additional testing.

Purpose of an Annual Physical Exam

A physical examination helps your PCP to determine the general status of your health.

The exam also gives you a chance to talk to them about any ongoing pain or symptoms that you're experiencing or any other health concerns that you might have.

A physical examination is recommended at least once a year, especially in people over the age of 50. These exams are used to:

- Check for possible diseases so they can be treated early,

- Identify any issues that may become medical concerns in the future,

- Update necessary immunizations,

- Ensure that you are maintaining a healthy diet and exercise routine, and

- Build a relationship with your PCP.

These exams are also a good way to check cholesterol, blood pressure, and blood sugar levels. These levels may be high without you ever showing any signs or symptoms. Regular screening allows your PCP to treat these conditions before they become severe.

Your PCP may also perform a physical exam before a surgery or before beginning your treatment for a medical condition.

Types

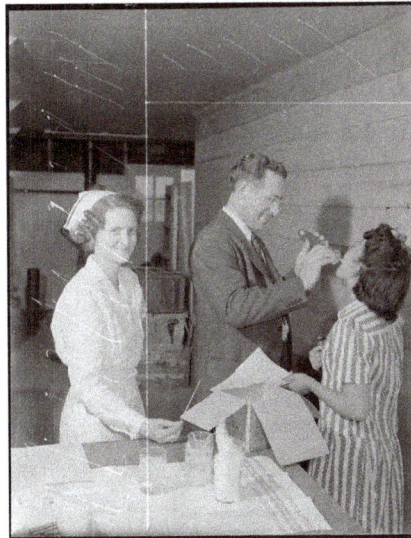

A resident physician, examining a patient's throat

Routine Physicals

Routine physicals are physical examinations performed on asymptomatic patients for medical screening purposes. These are normally performed by a pediatrician, family practice physician, physician assistant, a certified nurse practitioner or other primary care provider. This routine physical exam usually includes the HEENT evaluation. Nursing professionals such as registered nurse, licensed practical nurses develop a baseline assessment to identify normal versus abnormal findings. These are reported to the primary care provider.

Comprehensive Physicals

Comprehensive physical exams, also known as executive physicals, typically include laboratory tests, chest x-rays, pulmonary function testing, audiograms, full body CAT scanning, EKGs, heart stress tests, vascular age tests, urinalysis, and mammograms or prostate exams depending on gender.

Pre-employment Examinations

Pre-employment examinations are screening tests which judge the suitability of a worker for hire based on the results of their physical examination. This is also called *pre-employment medical clearance*. Many employers believe that by only hiring workers whose physical examination results pass certain exclusionary criteria, their employees collectively will have fewer absences due to sickness, fewer workplace injuries, and less occupational disease.

A small amount of low-quality evidence in medical research supports the idea that pre-employment physical examinations can actually reduce absences, workplace injuries, and occupational disease.

Employers should not routinely request that workers x-ray their lower backs as a condition for getting a job. Reasons for not doing this include the inability of such testing to predict future problems, the radiation exposure to the worker, and the cost of the exam.

Insurance Exams

These are physicals performed as a condition of buying health insurance or life insurance.

Uses

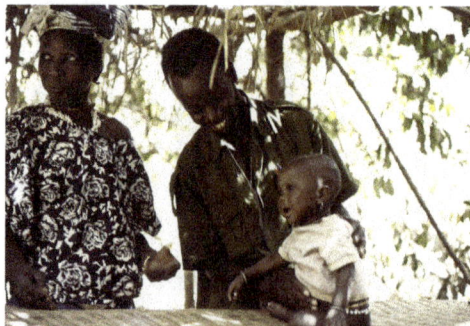

Medical doctor examines a young girl

Diagnosis

Physical examinations are performed in most healthcare encounters. For example, a physical examination is performed when a patient visits complaining of flu-like symptoms. These diagnostic examinations usually focus on the patient's chief complaint.

Screening

General health checks, including physical examinations performed when the patient reported no health concerns, often include medical screening for common conditions, such as high blood pressure. A Cochrane review found that general health checks did not reduce the risk of death from cancer, heart disease, or any other cause, and could not be proved to affect the patient's likelihood of being admitted to the hospital, becoming disabled, missing work, or needing additional office visits. The study found no effect on the risk of illness, but did find evidence suggesting that patients subject to routine physicals were diagnosed with hypertension and other chronic conditions at a higher rate than those who were not. Its authors noted that studies often failed to consider or report possible harmful outcomes (such as unwarranted anxiety or unnecessary follow-up procedures), and concluded that routine health checks were "unlikely to be beneficial" in regards to lowering cardiovascular and cancer morbidity and mortality.

Establishing Doctor-patient Relationship

In addition to the possibility of identifying signs of illness, it has been described as a ritual that plays a significant role in the doctor-patient relationship that will provide benefits in other medical encounters.

Format and Interpretation

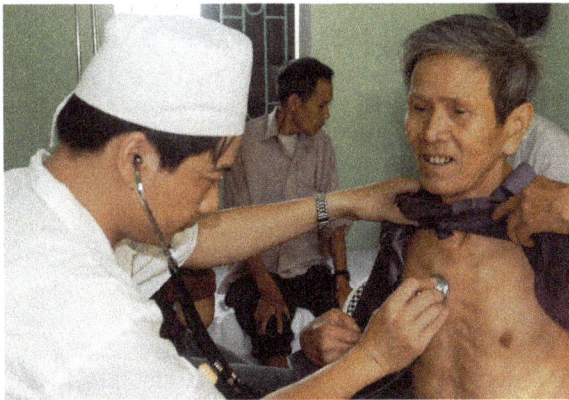

Auscultation of a man

A physical examination may include checking vital signs, including temperature examination, Blood pressure, pulse, and respiratory rate. The healthcare provider uses the senses of sight, hearing, touch, and sometimes smell (e.g., in infection, uremia, diabetic ketoacidosis). Taste has been made redundant by the availability of modern lab tests. Four actions are taught as the basis of physical examination: inspection, palpation (feel), percussion (tap to determine resonance characteristics), and auscultation (listen).

Check-up

While elective physical exams have become more elaborate, in routine use physical exams have become less complete. This has led to editorials in medical journals about the importance of an adequate physical examination.

Although providers have varying approaches as to the sequence of body parts, a systematic examination generally starts at the head and finishes at the extremities. After the main organ systems have been investigated by inspection, palpation, percussion, and auscultation, specific tests may follow (such as a neurological investigation, orthopedic examination) or specific tests when a particular disease is suspected (e.g. eliciting Trousseau's sign in hypocalcemia).

With the clues obtained during the *history* and *physical examination* the healthcare provider can now formulate a differential diagnosis, a list of potential causes of the symptoms. Specific diagnostic tests (or occasionally empirical therapy) generally confirm the cause, or shed light on other, previously overlooked, causes.

Physicians at Stanford University medical school have introduced a set of 25 key physical examination skills that were felt to be useful.

Example

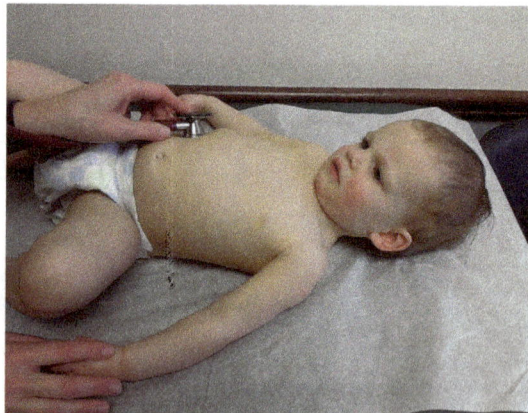

A doctor using a stethoscope to listen to a 15-month-old's abdomen

While the format of examination as listed below is largely as taught and expected of students, a specialist will focus on their particular field and the nature of the problem described by the patient. Hence a cardiologist will not in routine practice undertake neurological parts of the examination other than noting that the patient is able to use all four limbs on entering the consultation room and during the consultation become aware of their hearing, eyesight, and speech. Likewise an orthopaedic surgeon will examine the affected joint, but may only briefly check the heart sounds and chest to ensure that there is not likely to be any contraindication to surgery raised by the anaesthetist. A primary care physician will also generally examine the male genitals but may leave the examination of the female genitalia to a gynecologist.

A complete physical examination includes evaluation of general patient appearance and specific organ systems. It is recorded in the medical record in a standard layout which facilitates others later reading the notes. In practice the vital signs of temperature examination, pulse, and blood pressure are usually measured first.

Section	Sample text	Comments
General	"Patient in NAD. VS: WNL"	May be split on two lines. "WNL" = "within normal limits"
HEENT:	"NC/AT. PERRLA, EOMI. No cervical LAD, no thyromegaly, no bruit, no pallor, fundus WNL, oropharynx WNL, tympanic membrane WNL, neck supple"	"Neck" is sometimes split out from "Head". "Good dentition" may be noted.
Resp or "Chest"	"Nontender, CTA bilat" Chest expansion test, normal breathing with little effort, absence of wheezing, rhonchi and crackles.	More detailed examinations can include rales, rhonchi, wheezing ("no r/r/w"), and rubs. Other phrases may include "no cyanosis or clubbing" (if section is labeled "Resp" and not "Chest"), "fremitus WNL", and "no dullnes to percussion".
CV or "Heart"	"+S1, +S2, RRR, no m/r/g"	If "CV" is used instead of "heart", peripheral pulses are sometimes included in this section (otherwise, they may be in the extremities section)
Abd	"Soft, nontender, nondistended, absence of pain, no hepatosplenomegaly, NBS"	If lower back pain is involved, then the "Back" may become a primary section. Costovertebral angle tenderness may be included in the abdominal section if there is no back section. More detailed examinations may report "+psoas sign, +Rovsing's sign, +obturator sign". If tenderness was present, it might be reported as "Direct and rebound RLQ tenderness". "NBS" stands for "normal bowel sounds"; alternatives might include "hypoactive BS" or "hyperactive BS".
Ext	"No clubbing, cyanosis, edema"	Checking the fingers for clubbing and cyanosis is sometimes considered part of the pulmonary exam, because it closely involves oxygenation. Examinations of the knee may involve the McMurray test, Lachman test, and drawer test.
Neuro	"A&Ox3, CN II-XII grossly intact, Sensation intact in all four extremities (dull and sharp), DTR 2+ bilat, Romberg negative, cerebellar reflexes WNL, normal gait"	Sensation may be expanded to include dull, sharp, vibration, temperature, and position sense. A mental status exam may be reported at the beginning of the neurologic exam, or under a distinct "Psych" section.

Depending upon the chief complaint, additional sections may be included. For example, hearing may be evaluated with a specific Weber test and Rinne test, or it may be more briefly addressed in a cranial nerve exam. To give another example, a neurological related complaint might be evaluated with a specific test, such as the Romberg maneuver.

Head-to-toe Nursing Assessment

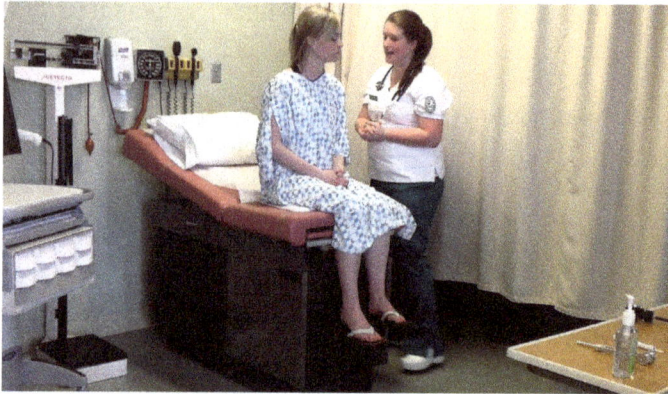

A comprehensive head-to-toe assessment is done on patient admission, at the beginning of each shift, and when it is determined to be necessary by the patient's hemodynamic status and the context. The head-to-toe assessment includes all the body systems, and the findings will inform the health care professional on the patient's overall condition. Any unusual findings should be followed up with a focused assessment specific to the affected body system.

Head-to-toe Assessment

Safety Considerations

- Perform hand hygiene.

- Check room for contact precautions.

- Introduce yourself to patient.

- Confirm patient ID using two patient identifiers (e.g., name and date of birth).

- Explain process to patient.

- Be organized and systematic in your assessment.

- Use appropriate listening and questioning skills.

- Listen and attend to patient cues.

- Ensure patient's privacy and dignity.

- Assess ABCCS (airway, breathing, circulation, consciousness, safety)/suction/ oxygen/safety.

- Apply principles of asepsis and safety.

- Check vital signs.

- Complete necessary focused assessments.

Steps

General Appearance

- Affect/behavior/anxiety

- Level of hygiene

- Body position

- Patient mobility

- Speech pattern and articulation.

Additional information:

Alterations may reflect neurologic impairment, oral injury or impairment, improperly fitting dentures, differences in dialect or language, or potential mental illness. Unusual findings should be followed up with a focused neurological system assessment.

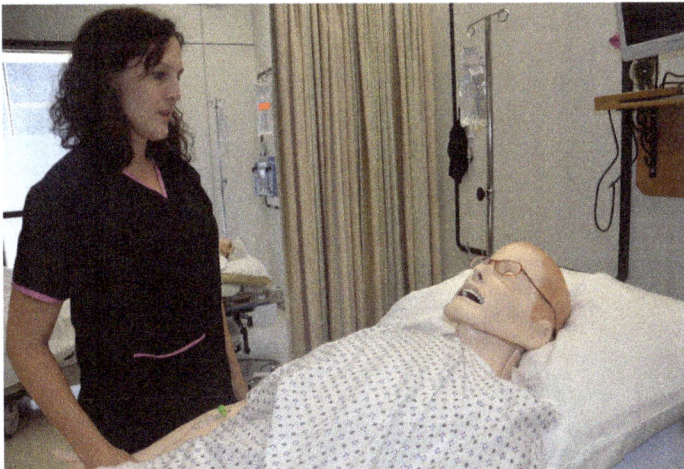

Assess general appearance

This is not a specific step. Evaluating the skin, hair, and nails is an ongoing element of a full body assessment.

Skin, Hair and Nails

- Inspect for lesions, bruising, and rashes.

- Palpate skin for temperature, moisture and texture.

- Inspect for pressure areas.

- Inspect skin for edema.

- Inspect scalp for lesions and hair and scalp for presence of lice and/or nits.

- Inspect nails for consistency, color, and capillary refill.

Additional information:

Check for and follow up on the presence of lesions, bruising, and rashes. Variations in skin temperature, texture, and perspiration or dehydration may indicate underlying conditions.

Redness of the skin at pressure areas such as heels, elbows, buttocks, and hips indicates the need to reassess patient's need for position changes.

Unilateral edema may indicate a local or peripheral cause, whereas bilateral-pitting edema usually indicates cardiac or kidney failure.

Check hair for the presence of lice and/or nits (eggs), which are oval in shape and adhere to the hair shaft.

Head and Neck

- Inspect eyes for drainage.

- Inspect eyes for pupillary reaction to light.

- Inspect mouth, tongue, and teeth for moisture, color, dentures.

- Inspect for facial symmetry.

Additional information:

Check eyes for drainage, pupil size, and reaction to light. Drainage may indicate infection, allergy, or injury.

Slow pupillary reaction to light or unequal reactions bilaterally may indicate neurological impairment.

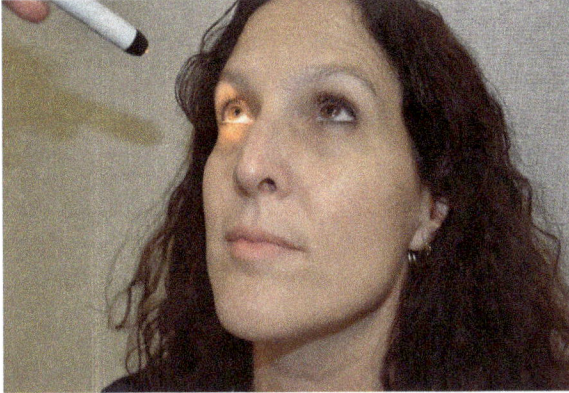

Check pupillary reaction to light

Dry mucous membranes indicate decreased hydration.

Facial asymmetry may indicate neurological impairment or injury. Unusual findings should be followed up with a focused neurological system assessment.

Chest

- Inspect:

  - Expansion/retraction of chest wall/work of breathing and/or accessory muscle use

  - Jugular distension.

- Auscultate:

  - For breath sounds anteriorly and posteriorly

  - Apices and bases for any adventitious sounds

  - Apical heart rate.

- Palpate:

  - For symmetrical lung expansion.

Additional information:

Chest expansion may be asymmetrical with conditions such as atelectasis, pneumonia, fractured ribs, or pneumothorax.

Use of accessory muscles may indicate acute airway obstruction or massive atelectasis. Jugular distension of more than 3 cm above the sternal angle while the patient is at 45° may indicate cardiac failure.

The presence of crackles or wheezing must be further assessed, documented, and reported. Unusual findings should be followed up with a focused respiratory assessment.

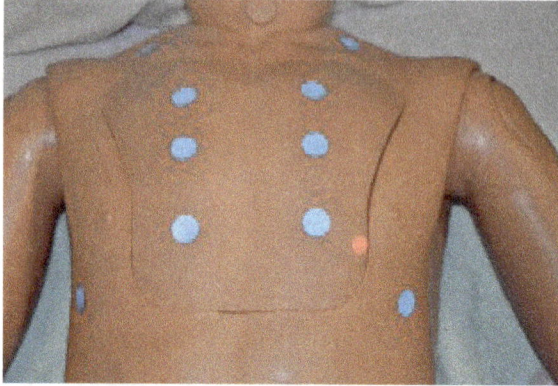

Auscultate anterior chest; blue dots indicate stethoscope placement for auscultation

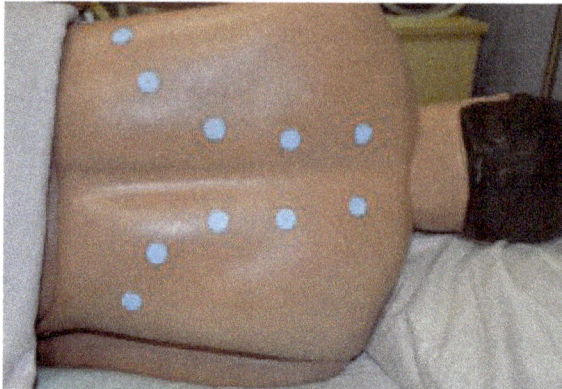

Auscultate posterior chest; blue dots indicate stethoscope placement for auscultation

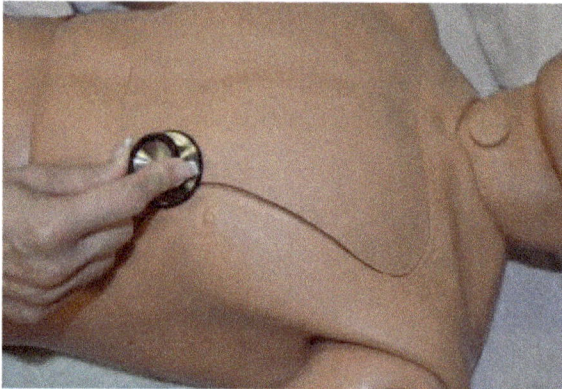

Auscultate apical pulse at the fifth intercostal space and midclavicular line

Note the heart rate and rhythm, identify S1 and S2, and follow up on any unusual findings with a focused cardiovascular assessment.

Abdomen

- Inspect:

    ○ Abdomen for distension, asymmetry.

- Auscultate:

  - Bowel sounds (RLQ).

- Palpate:

  - Four quadrants for pain and bladder/bowel distension (light palpation only).

- Check urine output for frequency, color, odour.

- Determine frequency and type of bowel movements.

Additional information:

Abdominal distension may indicate ascites associated with conditions such as heart failure, cirrhosis, and pancreatitis. Markedly visible peristalsis with abdominal distension may indicate intestinal obstruction.

Hyperactive bowel sounds may indicate bowel obstruction, gastroenteritis, or subsiding paralytic ileum.

Hypoactive or absent bowel sounds may be present after abdominal surgery, or with peritonitis or paralytic ileus.

Pain and tenderness may indicate underlying inflammatory conditions such as peritonitis.

Unusual findings in urine output may indicate compromised urinary function. Follow up with a focused gastrointestinal and genitourinary assessment.

Unusual findings with bowel movements should be followed up with a focused gastrointestinal and genitourinary assessment.

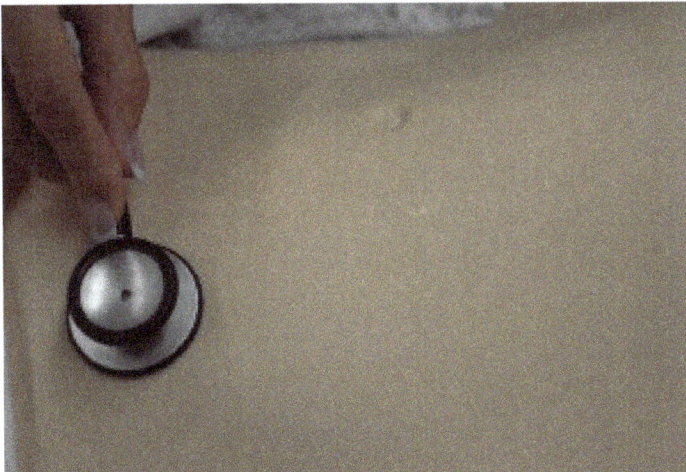

Auscultate abdomen

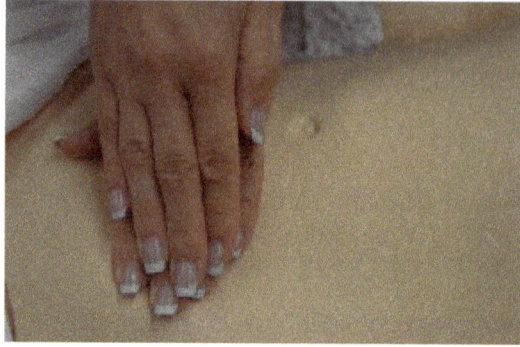

Palpate abdomen

Extremities

- Inspect:

  - Arms and legs for pain, deformity, edema, pressure areas, bruises

  - Compare bilaterally

- Palpate:

  - Radial pulses

  - Pedal pulses: dorsalis pedis and posterior tibial

  - CWMS and capillary refill (hands and feet)

- Assess handgrip strength and equality.

- Assess dorsiflex and plantarflex feet against resistance (note strength and equality).

- Check skin integrity and pressure areas.

Additional information:

Limitation in range of movement may indicate articular disease or injury.

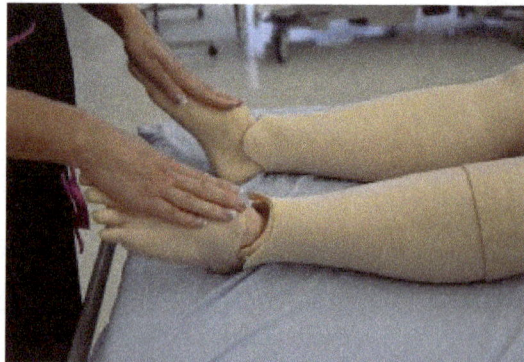

Assess plantar flexion

Palpate pulses for symmetry in rate and rhythm. Asymmetry may indicate cardiovascular conditions or post-surgical complications.

Unequal handgrip and/or foot strength may indicate underlying conditions, injury, or post-surgical complications.

CWMS: color, warmth, movement, and sensation of the hands and feet should be checked and compared to determine adequacy of perfusion.

Check skin integrity and pressure areas, and ensure follow-up and in-depth assessment of patient mobility and need for regular changes in position.

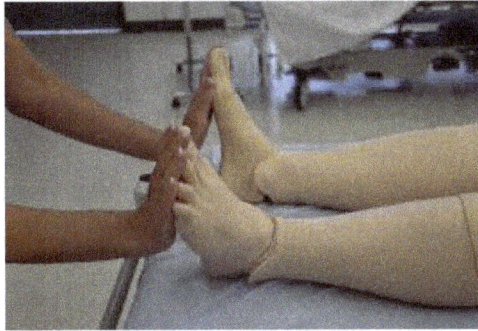

Assess dorsiflexion

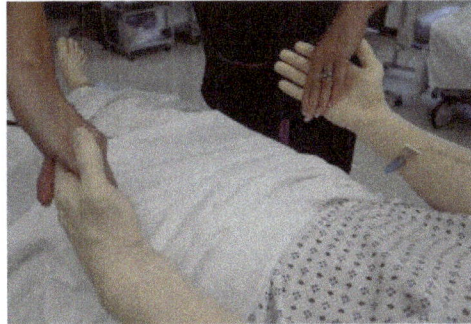

Assess bilateral hand strength

Palpate and inspect capillary refill and report if more than 3 seconds.

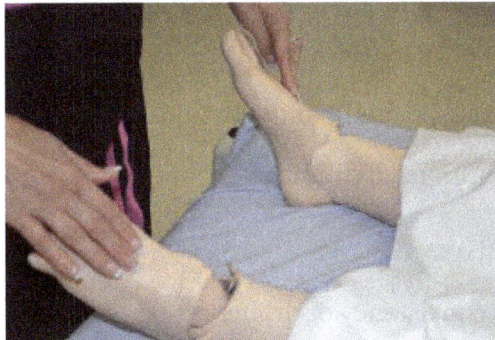

Assess pedal pulses

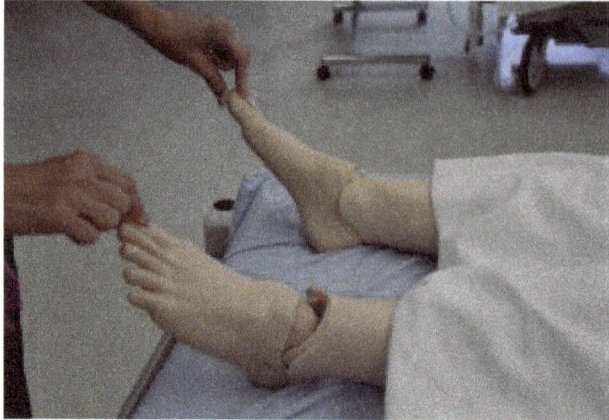

Check capillary refill

To check capillary refill, depress the nail edge to cause blanching and then release. Color should return to the nail instantly or in less than 3 seconds. If it takes longer, this suggests decreased peripheral perfusion and may indicate cardiovascular or respiratory dysfunction. Unusual findings should be followed up with a focused cardiovascular assessment.

Clubbing of nails, in which the nails present as straightened out to 180 degrees, with the nail base feeling spongy, occurs with heart disease, emphysema, and chronic bronchitis.

Back Area (Turn Patient to side or ask to Sit up or Lean Forward)

- Inspect back and spine.

- Inspect coccyx/buttocks.

Additional information:

Check for curvature or abnormalities in the spine.

Check skin integrity and pressure areas, and ensure follow-up and in-depth assessment of patient mobility and need for regular changes in position.

Tubes, Drains, Dressings and IVs

- Inspect for drainage, position, and function.

- Assess wounds for unusual drainage.

Additional Information

Note amount, color, and consistency of drainage (e.g., Foley catheter), or if infusing as prescribed (e.g., intravenous).

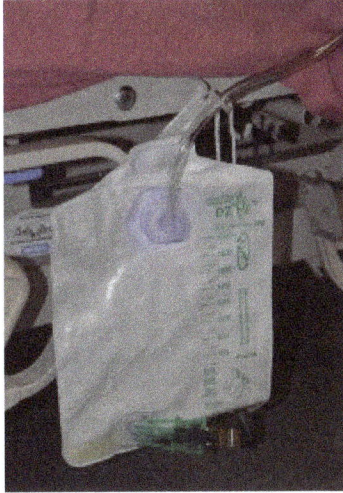

Urinary catheter bag

Assess wounds for large amounts of drainage or for purulent drainage, and provide wound care as indicated.

Mobility

- Check if full or partial weight-bearing.

- Determine gait/balance.

- Determine need for and use of assistive devices.

Additional information:

Assess patient's risk for falls. Document and follow up any indication of falls risk. Note use of mobility aids and ensure they are available to the patient on ambulation.

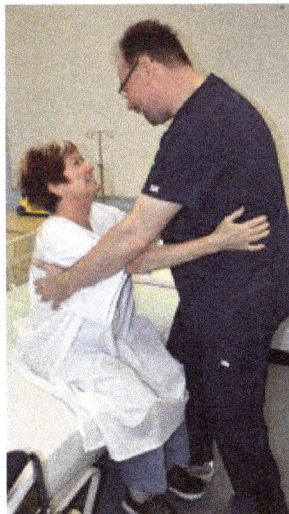

Patient position prior to standing

Report and document assessment findings and related health problems according to agency policy.

Accurate and timely documentation and reporting promote patient safety.

References

- Verghese A, Horwitz RI (2009). "In praise of the physical examination" (PDF). BMJ. 339: b5448. doi:10.1136/bmj.b5448. PMID 20015910

- Physical-examination, health: healthline.com, Retrieved 27 May 2018

- Flegel KM (November 1999). "Does the physical examination have a future?". Canadian Medical Association Journal. 161 (9): 1117–8. PMC 1230732. PMID 10569087

- Natt, B; Szerlip, HM (2014), "The lost art of the history and physical", Am J Med Sci, 348(5): 423–425, doi:10.1097/MAJ.0000000000000326, PMID 25247755

- 2-2-head-to-toe-assessment-checklist: opentextbc.ca, Retrieved 19 June 2018

- Armour, Lawrence A. (21 July 1997). "2,500 executives flock to Rochester, Minn., for a deluxe, soup-to-nuts physical at the Mayo clinic. Our man went for a tune-up to find out why". CNN.com. Retrieved 16 July 2009

Activities of Daily Living (ADLs)

Activities of daily living(ADLs) refer to the daily self-care activities of a person. The assessment of ADLs in individuals post an injury or trauma, or suffering from a disability or age, allows information regarding their functional status. In order to completely understand activities of daily living, it is necessary to understand the processes related to it. The following chapter elucidates the varied processes and mechanisms associated with this area of study.

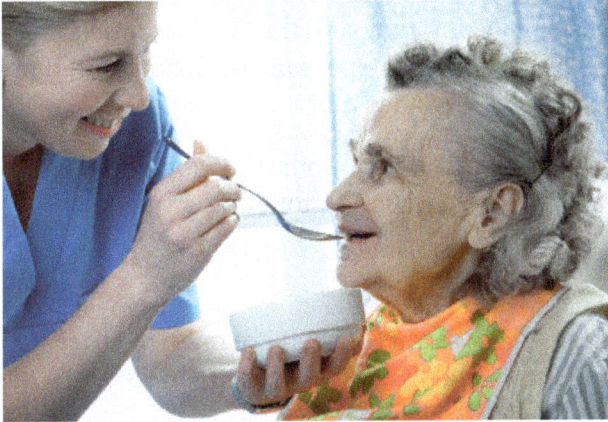

Activities of daily living are activities related to personal care. They include bathing or showering, dressing, getting in and out of bed or a chair, walking, using the toilet, and eating. If a sample person has difficulty performing an activity by himself/herself and without special equipment, or does not perform the activity at all because of health problems, the person is deemed to have a limitation in that activity. The limitation may be temporary or chronic at the time of the survey. Sample persons who are administered a community interview answer health status and functioning questions themselves, unless they are unable to do so. A proxy, such as a nurse, always answers questions about the sample person's health status and functioning for long-term care facility interviews.

Basic ADLs consist of self-care tasks that include, but are not limited to:

- Bathing and showering.

- Personal hygiene and grooming (including brushing/combing/styling hair).

- Dressing.

- Toilet hygiene (getting to the toilet, cleaning oneself, and getting back up).

- Functional mobility, often referred to as "transferring", as measured by the ability to walk, get in and out of bed, and get into and out of a chair; the broader definition (moving from one place to another while performing activities) is useful for people with different physical abilities who are still able to get around independently.

- Self-feeding (not including cooking or chewing and swallowing).

One way to think about basic ADLs is that they are the things many people do when they get up in the morning and get ready to go out of the house: get out of bed, go to the toilet, bathe, dress, groom, and eat.

There is a hierarchy to the ADLs: "… the early loss function is hygiene, the mid-loss functions are toilet use and locomotion, and the late loss function is eating. When there is only one remaining area in which the person is independent, there is a 62.9% chance that it is eating and only a 3.5% chance that it is hygiene."

Although not in wide general use, a mnemonic that some find useful is DEATH: dressing/bathing, eating, ambulating (walking), toileting, hygiene.

Instrumental

Instrumental activities of daily living (IADLs) are not necessary for fundamental functioning, but they let an individual live independently in a community:

- Cleaning and maintaining the house

- Managing money

- Moving within the community

- Preparing meals

- Shopping for groceries and necessities

- Taking prescribed medications

- Using the telephone or other form of communication.

Occupational therapists often evaluate IADLs when completing patient assessments. The American Occupational Therapy Association identifies 12 types of IADLs that may be performed as a co-occupation with others:

- Care of others (including selecting and supervising caregivers)

- Care of pets

- Child rearing

- Communication management

- Community mobility

- Financial management

- Health management and maintenance

- Home establishment and maintenance

- Meal preparation and cleanup

- Religious observances

- Safety procedures and emergency responses

- Shopping.

Role of Therapy

Occupational therapists teach and rebuild the skills required to maintain, regain or increase a person's independence in all Activities of Daily Living that have declined because of health conditions (physical or mental), injury or age-related debility.

Physical therapists use exercises to assist patients in maintaining and gaining independence in ADLs. The exercise program is based on what components patients are lacking such as walking speed, strength, balance, and coordination. Slow walking speed is associated with increased risk of falls. Exercise enhances walking speed, allowing for safer and more functional ambulation capabilities. After initiating an exercise program it is important to maintain the routine otherwise the benefits will be lost. Exercise for patients who are frail is essential for preserving functional independence and avoiding the necessity for care from others or placement in a long term care facility.

Assistance

Assisting in activities of daily living are skills required in nursing and as well as other professions such as nursing assistants. This includes assisting in patient mobility, such as moving an activity intolerant patient within bed. For hygiene, this often involves bed baths and assisting with urinary and bowel elimination.

Evaluation

There are several evaluation tools, such as the Katz ADL scale, the Older Americans Resources and Services (OARS) ADL/IADL scale, the Lawton IADL scale and the Bristol Activities of Daily Living Scale.

In the domain of disability, measures have been developed to capture functional recovery in performing basic activities of daily living. Among them, some measures like the Functional Independence Measure are designed for assessment across a wide range of disabilities. Others like the Spinal Cord Independence Measure are designed to evaluate participants in a specific type of disability.

Most models of health care service use ADL evaluations in their practice, including the medical (or institutional) models, such as the Roper-Logan-Tierney model of nursing, and the resident-centered models, such as the Program of All-Inclusive Care for the Elderly (PACE).

Instrumental Activities of Daily Living

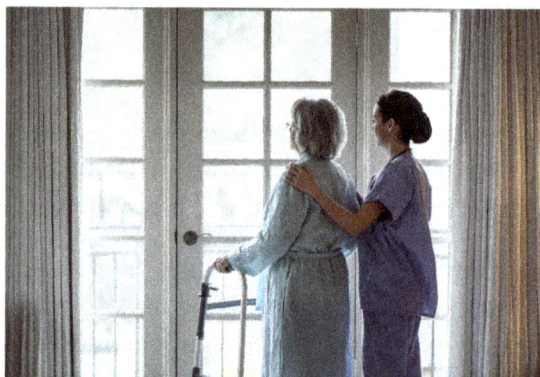

These are the self-care tasks we usually learn as teenagers. They require more complex thinking skills, including organizational skills. They include:

- Managing finances, such as paying bills and managing financial assets.

- Managing transportation, either via driving or by organizing other means of transport.

- Shopping and meal preparation. This covers everything required to get a meal on the table. It also covers shopping for clothing and other items required for daily life.

- Housecleaning and home maintenance. This means cleaning kitchens after eating, keeping one's living space reasonably clean and tidy, and keeping up with home maintenance.

- Managing communication, such as the telephone and mail.

- Managing medications, which covers obtaining medications and taking them as directed.

References

- Williams, Brie (2014). "Consideration of Function & Functional Decline". Current Diagnosis and Treatment: Geriatrics, Second Edition. New York, NY: McGraw-Hill. pp. 3–4. ISBN 978-0-07-179208-0

- Research-statistics-data-and-systems: cms.gov, Retrieved 17 July 2018

- Morris, John M. ""Scaling functional status within the interRAI suite of assessment instruments" John". Retrieved 9 March 2017

- Alexander, MS (2009). "Outcome measures in spinal cord injury : recent assessments and recommendations for future directions". Spinal cord. doi:10.1038/sc.2009.18

- What-are-adls-and-iadls: betterhealthwhileaging.net, Retrieved 28 May 2018

- Gurland, Barry J.; Maurer, Mathew S. "Life and Works of Sidney Katz, MD: A Life Marked by Fundamental Discovery". Journal of the American Medical Directors Association. 13(9): 764–65. doi:10.1016/j.jamda.2012.09.003

Medication Administration

The administration of medication to people suffering from a disease or diseases falls in the domain of medication administration. This chapter discusses in detail the diverse aspects and procedures involved in medication administration, such as rights and routes of medication administration.

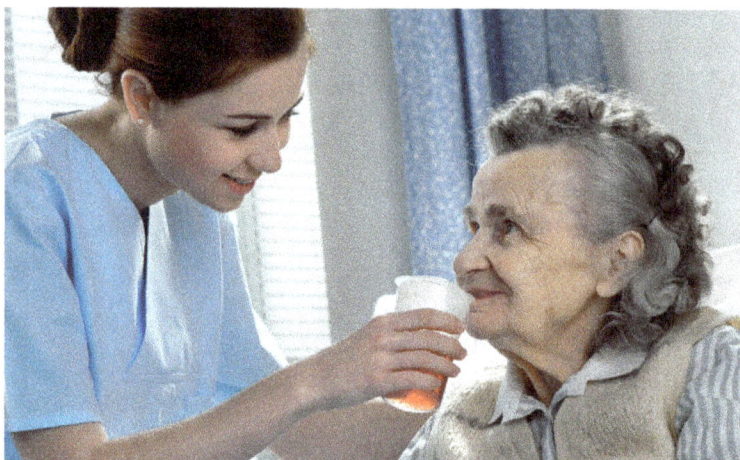

The administration of medication to a patient is often a chief responsibility of the nurse. The practice of administering medication involves providing the patient with a substance prescribed and intended for the diagnosis, treatment, or prevention of a medical illness or condition.

The central action of medication administration involves actual and complete conveyance of a medication to the patient. However, there is a wider set of practices required to achieve safe, effective patient outcomes and to prepare for and evaluate the outcome of medication administration.

Laws regarding medication administration vary from state to state. Doctors, physicians, physician assistants, nurse practitioners, and nurses are generally trained and authorized to administer medication, while other medical disciplines may have a limited responsibility in this area. In certain circumstances, unlicensed personnel may be trained and authorized to administer medication in residential care settings. State and federal laws also restrict the distribution of and access to medications that can be abused (called controlled substances). Responsibility for controlled substances includes accountability for any discarded substances, double-locked storage, and counting of medication supply at regular intervals by clinician teams.

Preparation for medication administration begins with the order for medication, in most circumstances written by the physician. and physician assistants are also often authorized to write prescriptions. State laws vary regarding these privileges. A record of orders for medication and other treatments is kept in the medical chart. Universally accepted safe clinical practice guidelines and state laws govern the components of medication orders in order to ensure consistency and patient safety. All orders should contain the patient's name, the date and time when the order is written, and the signature of the ordering clinician. Care givers administering medication are responsible for checking that these components are present and clear. The name of the medication is accompanied by the dosage, or how much of the drug should be given; the route of administration, or how the medication should be given (i.e., intramuscular injection); and frequency, or how often the drug is to be given.

Rights of Medication Administration

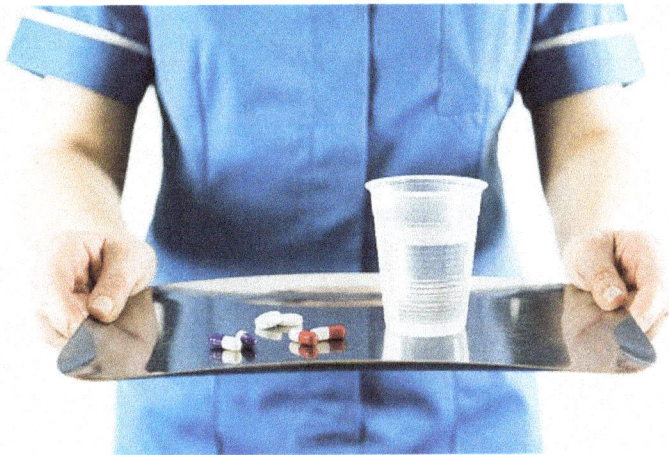

Right Patient

- Check the name on the order and the patient.

- Use 2 identifiers.

- Ask patient to identify himself/herself.

- When available, use technology (for example, bar-code system).

Right Medication

- Check the medication label.

- Check the order.

Right Dose

- Check the order.

- Confirm appropriateness of the dose using a current drug reference.

- If necessary, calculate the dose and have another nurse calculate the dose as well.

Right Route

- Again, check the order and appropriateness of the route ordered.

- Confirm that the patient can take or receive the medication by the ordered route.

Right Time

- Check the frequency of the ordered medication.

- Double-check that you are giving the ordered dose at the correct time.

- Confirm when the last dose was given.

Right Documentation

- Document administration AFTER giving the ordered medication.

- Chart the time, route, and any other specific information as necessary. For example, the site of an injection or any laboratory value or vital sign that needed to be checked before giving the drug.

Right Reason

- Confirm the rationale for the ordered medication. What is the patient's history? Why is he/she taking this medication?

- Revisit the reasons for long-term medication use.

Right Response

- Make sure that the drug led to the desired effect. If an antihypertensive was given, has his/her blood pressure improved? Does the patient verbalize improvement in depression while on an antidepressant?

- Be sure to document your monitoring of the patient and any other nursing interventions that are applicable.

Routes of Medication Administration

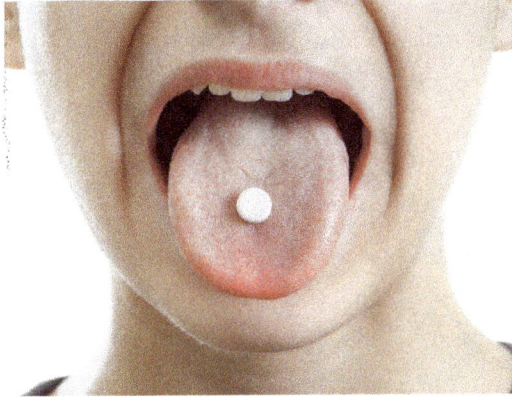

Route	Explanation
Buccal	held inside the cheek
Enteral	delivered directly into the stomach or intestine (with a G-tube or J-tube)
Inhalable	breathed in through a tube or mask
Infused	injected into a vein with an IV line and slowly dripped in over time
Intramuscular	injected into muscle with a syringe
Intrathecal	injected into your spine
Intravenous	injected into a vein or into an IV line
Nasal	given into the nose by spray or pump
Ophthalmic	given into the eye by drops, gel, or ointment
Oral	swallowed by mouth as a tablet, capsule, lozenge, or liquid
Otic	given by drops into the ear
Rectal	inserted into the rectum
Subcutaneous	injected just under the skin
Sublingual	held under the tongue
Topical	applied to the skin
Transdermal	given through a patch placed on the skin

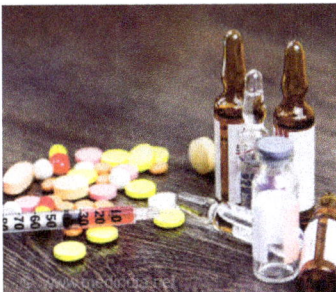

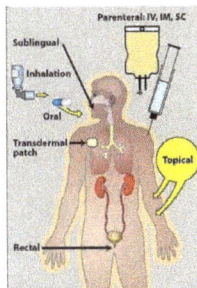

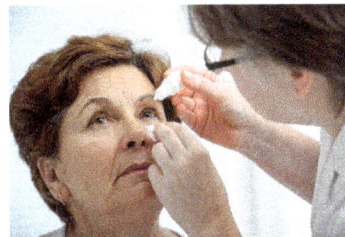

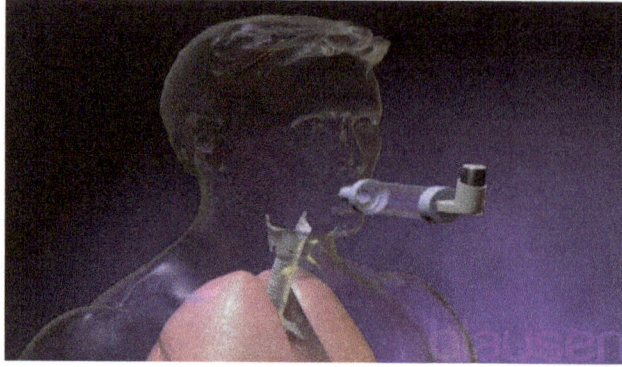

Pain Management

The interdisciplinary branch of medicine that uses different approaches to ease the suffering and improve a person's quality of life is known as pain management. This chapter explores the fundamentals and practices of interventional pain management, acupuncture, transcutaneous electrical nerve stimulation, etc.

Pain management is the process of providing medical care that alleviates or reduces pain. Mild to moderate pain can usually be treated with analgesic medications, such as aspirin. For chronic or severe pain, opiates and other narcotics may be used, sometimes in concert with analgesics; with steroids or nonsteroidal anti-inflammatory drugs when the pain is related to inflammation; or with antidepressants, which can potentiate some pain medications without raising the actual dose of the drug and which affect the brain's perception of pain. Narcotics carry with them the potential for side effects and addiction. However, the risk of addiction is not normally a concern in the care of terminal patients. For hospitalized patients with severe pain, devices for self-administration of narcotics are frequently used. Other procedures can also be useful in pain management programs. For bedridden patients, simply changing position regularly or using pillows to support a more comfortable posture can be effective. Massage, acupuncture, acupressure, and biofeedback have also shown some validity for increased pain control in some patients.

Pain management can be simple or complex, depending on the cause of the pain. An example of pain that is typically less complex would be nerve root irritation from a herniated disc with pain radiating down the leg. This condition can often be alleviated with an epidural steroid injection and physical therapy. Sometimes, however, the pain does not go away. This can require a wide variety of skills and techniques to treat the pain. These skills and techniques include:

- Interventional procedures;
- Medication management;
- Physical therapy or chiropractic therapy;
- Psychological counseling and support;
- Acupuncture and other alternative therapies; and
- Referral to other medical specialists.

All of these skills and services are necessary because pain can involve many aspects of a person's daily life.

Physical Medicine and Rehabilitation

Physical Medicine and Rehabilitation (PM&R), also known as physiatry, is a medical specialty that involves restoring function for a person who has been disabled as a result of a disease, disorder, or injury.

Physiatry provides integrated, multidisciplinary care aimed at recovery of the whole person by addressing the individual's physical, emotional, medical, vocational, and social needs. A doctor who specializes in physical medicine and rehabilitation is called a physiatrist.

Rehabilitation

Rehabilitation is the process of helping a person achieve the highest level of function, independence, and quality of life possible. Rehab does not reverse or undo the damage caused by disease or injury, but rather helps restore the person to optimal health, functioning, and well-being. Rehabilitate means to make able.

Rehabilitation Program

Rehabilitation medicine is designed to meet each person's specific needs; therefore, each program is different. Some general treatment components for rehab programs include:

- Treating the basic disease and preventing complications

- Treating the disability and improving function

- Providing adaptive tools and altering the environment

- Teaching the patient and family and helping them adapt to lifestyle changes.

The success of rehab depends on many variables, including:

- The nature and severity of the disease, disorder, or injury

- The type and degree of any resulting impairments and disabilities

- The overall health of the patient

- Family support.

Areas covered in rehabilitation programs may include the following:

Patient need	Example
Self-care skills, including activities of daily living (ADLs)	Feeding, grooming, bathing, dressing, toileting, and sexual function
Physical care	Nutritional needs, medicine, and skin care
Mobility skills	Walking, transfers, and self-propelling a wheelchair
Respiratory care	Ventilator care, if needed; breathing treatments and exercises to promote lung function
Communication skills	Speech, writing, and alternative methods of communication
Cognitive skills	Memory, concentration, judgment, problem solving, and organizational skills
Socialization skills	Interacting with others at home and within the community
Vocational training	Work-related skills
Pain management	Medicine and alternative methods of managing pain
Psychological counseling	Identifying problems and solutions with thinking, behavioral, and emotional issues
Family support	Assistance with adapting to lifestyle changes, financial concerns, and discharge planning
Education	Patient and family education and training about the condition, medical care, and adaptive techniques

Rehabilitation is needed when a disease and injury causes an impairment. Consider the following:

- An impairment is a loss of normal function of part of the body, such as paralysis of a leg.

- Disability occurs when a person is not able to perform an activity in a normal way as a result of an impairment, such as not being able to walk.

- A handicap occurs when there are limits that prevent a person with a disability from performing a role that is normal for that person, such as not being able to work. A handicap refers to a barrier that may be imposed by society, the environment, or by one's own attitude.

Most people with disabilities are not considered handicapped. They go to school, work, perform family duties, and interact with society fully and capably.

Transcutaneous Electrical Nerve Stimulation

One of the most common forms of electrical stimulation used for pain management is transcutaneous electrical nerve stimulation (TENS) therapy, which provides short-term pain relief. Electrical nerve stimulation and electrothermal therapy are used to relieve pain associated with various conditions, including back pain. Intradiscal electrothermal therapy (IDET) is a treatment option for people with low back pain resulting from intervertebral disc problems.

TENS Therapy for Pain Management

In TENS therapy for pain management, a small, battery-operated device delivers low-voltage electrical current through the skin via electrodes placed near the source of pain. The electricity from the electrodes stimulates nerves in the affected area and sends signals to the brain that "scramble" normal pain perception. TENS is not painful and may be effective therapy to mask pain such as diabetic neuropathy. However, TENS for chronic low back pain is not effective and cannot be recommended, the American Academy of Neurology (AAN) now says.

Intradiscal Electrothermal Therapy (IDET)

Intervertebral discs act as cushions between the vertebrae. Sometimes the discs can become damaged and cause pain. IDET uses heat to modify the nerve fibers of a spinal disc and to destroy pain receptors in the area. In this procedure, a wire called an electrothermal catheter is placed through an incision in the disc. An electrical current passes through the wire, heating a small outer portion of the disc to a temperature of 90 degrees Celsius. IDET is performed as an outpatient procedure while the patient is awake and under a local anesthesia.

Early studies indicated that some patients may have continued pain relief for up to six months or longer. The long-term effects of this procedure on the disc, however, have not been determined. More studies are needed to compare this treatment to standard therapies and surgery as well as placebo.

Radiofrequency Discal Nucleoplasty

Radiofrequency discal nucleoplasty is a newer procedure which utilizes a radio frequency probe instead of heating wire to disintegrate a small portion of the central disc material. The result of this intervention is partial decompression of the disc, which may help relieve pain caused by bulging discs pressing on nearby spinal nerve roots.

Acupuncture

Acupuncture is a form of treatment that involves inserting very thin needles through a person's skin at specific points on the body, to various depths.

Research suggests that it can help relieve pain, and it is used for a wide range of other complaints.

However, according to the National Center for Complementary and Integrative Health (NCCIH), there is limited evidence for its effectiveness in areas other than pain.

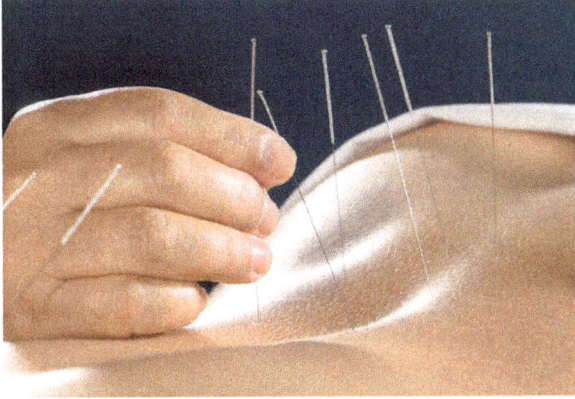

How acupuncture works scientifically remains unclear. Some people claim it works by balancing vital energy, while others believe it has a neurological effect

Acupuncture remains controversial among Western medical doctors and scientists.

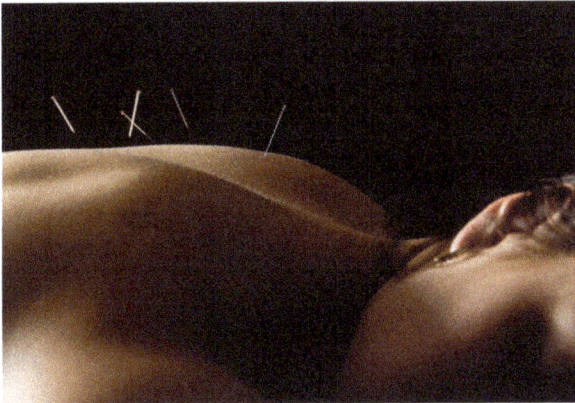

Acupuncture involves inserting needles at certain points of the body

An acupuncurist will insert needles into a person's body with the aim of balancing their energy.

This, it is claimed, can help boost wellbeing and may cure some illnesses.

Conditions it is used for include different kinds of pain, such as headaches, blood pressureproblems, and whooping cough, among others.

Working of Acupuncture

Traditional Chinese medicine explains that health is the result of a harmonious balance of the complementary extremes of "yin" and "yang" of the life force known as "qi," pronounced "chi." Illness is said to be the consequence of an imbalance of the forces.

Qi is said to flow through meridians, or pathways, in the human body. These meridiens and energy flows are accessible through 350 acupuncture points in the body.

Inserting needles into these points with appropriate combinations is said to bring the energy flow back into proper balance.

There is no scientific proof that the meridians or acupuncture points exist, and it is hard to prove that they either do or do not, but numerous studies suggest that acupuncture works for some conditions.

Some experts have used neuroscience to explain acupuncture. Acupuncture points are seen as places where nerves, muscles, and connective tissue can be stimulated. The stimulation increases blood flow, while at the same time triggering the activity of the body›s natural painkillers.

It is difficult to set up investigations using proper scientific controls, because of the invasive nature of acupuncture. In a clinical study, a control group would have to undergo sham treatment, or a placebo, for results to be compared with those of genuine acupuncture.

Some studies have concluded that acupuncture offers similar benefits to a patient as a placebo, but others have indicated that there are some real benefits.

Uses

Research carried out in Germany has shown that acupuncture may help relieve tension headaches and migraines.

The NCCIH note that it has been proven to help in cases of:

- Low back pain

- Neck pain

- Osteoarthritis

- Knee pain

- Headache and migraine.

They list additional disorders that may benefit from acupuncture, but which require further scientific confirmation.

In 2003, the World Health Organization (WHO) listed a number of conditions in which they say acupuncture has been proven effective.

These include:

- High and low blood pressure

- Chemotherapy-induced nausea and vomiting

- Some gastric conditions, including peptic ulcer

- Painful periods

- Dysentery

- Allergic rhinitis

- Facial pain

- Morning sickness

- Rheumatoid arthritis

- Sprains

- Tennis elbow

- Sciatica

- Dental pain

- Reducing the risk of stroke

- Inducing labor.

Other conditions for which the WHO say that acupuncture may help but more evidence is needed include:

- Fibromyalgia

- Neuralgia

- Post-operative convalescence

- Substance, tobaccor and alcohol dependence

- Spine pain

- Stiff neck

- Vascular dementia

- Whooping cough, or pertussis

- Tourette syndrome.

The WHO also suggest that it may help treat a number of infections, including some urinary tract infections and epidemic hemorrhagic fever.

They point out, however, that "only national health authorities can determine the diseases, symptoms, and conditions for which acupuncture treatment can be recommended."

Benefits

Acupuncture can be beneficial in that:

- Performed correctly, it is safe.

- There are very few side effects.

- It can be effectively combined with other treatments.

- It can control some types of pain.

- It may help patients for whom pain medications are not suitable.

The NCCIH advise people not to use acupuncture instead of seeing a conventional health care provider.

Interventional Pain Management

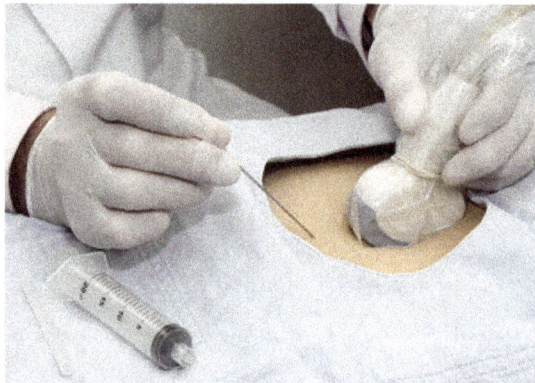

Interventional pain management is a method which utilizes pain blocking techniques to help make day-to-day activities less difficult, and effectively restore quality of life for patients. Surgery, electrostimulation, nerve blocks or implantable drug delivery systems may be used as part of the treatment process.

Interventional pain management is generally used when pain is severe enough to interfere with daily activities, and other treatment types have not been successful in reducing pain. If you are searching for a solution to your chronic or acute pain, then it may be time to find an Interventional Pain Management doctor who can help.

Types of Interventional Pain Management Treatments

There are many types of interventional pain management treatments. The type of treatment you receive will be based on your specific condition and symptoms, as each type of treatment varies in terms of invasiveness. Some of the most common lnterventional pain management techniques include:

- Nerve Blocks: Pain signals travel down nerves to the brain. Nerve blocks are used to interrupt these signals to provide pain relief. The type of nerve block depends will depend on your treatment plan, as some are minimally invasive and may last for hours or days. Other nerve blocks require surgical procedures, and may be long-term or permanent.

- Infusions: Infusions involve the delivery of pain relief drugs directly into the body. These are generally for longer-term use. intrathecal infusions are delivered into the subarachnoid space in the brain; epidural infusions are used in the spinal cord.

- Injections: Some common types of injections are Epidural Steroid Injections, Facet Joint Injections and Trigger Joint Injections. Each of these injections target different pain spots in the body. Injections generally include a numbing agent and a steroid.

- Radiofrequency Ablation: This treatment is usually used to treat lower back and neck pain, especially when pain is caused by arthritis. This technique uses a radio wave to produce an electrical current, which is then used to heat an area of nerve tissue. This method decreases the pain signals from that area.

- Spinal Cord Stimulation: This technique treats chronic pain by applying gentle electrical currents to the source of the pain. Electrical leads are inserted close to the spinal column, while a tiny generator is inserted into the abdomen or buttock. The generator emits electrical signals to the spinal column, thus blocking the ability for the brain to perceive pain.

- Peripheral Nerve Field Stimulation: This treatment type is related to Spinal Cord Stimulation, except that it is localized on other parts of the body. The electrical leads are placed as close to the source of pain as possible and follows the same general process as spinal cord stimulation.

References

- Health-library, physical-medicine-and-rehabilitation, overview-of-physical-medicine-and-rehabilitation-pmr-85: hopkinsmedicine.org, Retrieved 17 April 2018

- Pain-management: medicinenet.com, Retrieved 16 May 2018

- Electrothermal-therapy, back-pain: webmd.com, Retrieved 09 July 2018

- What-is-interventional-pain-management: floridamedicalclinic.com, Retrieved 28 May 2018

End-of-life Care

End-of-life care is the health care of a terminally ill person when the medical condition in its advanced stage, or of any individual in the final hours or days of his life. This chapter has been carefully written to provide an understanding of nursing care to a person near death. It includes the topics like palliative care, hospice care and spiritual care.

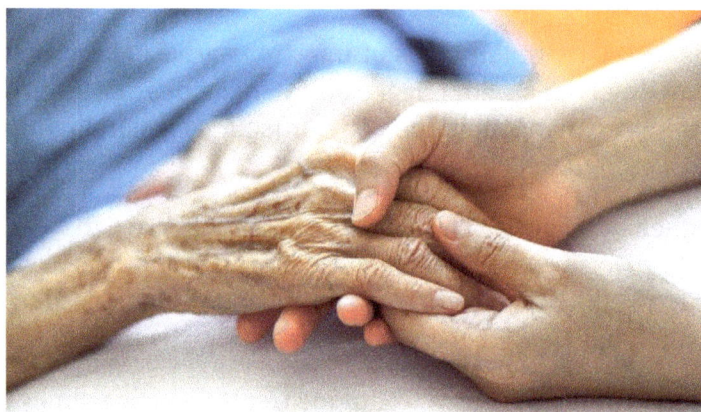

End of life care is support for people who are in the last months or years of their life

End of life care should help you to live as well as possible until you die and to die with dignity. The people providing your care should ask you about your wishes and preferences, and take these into account as they work with you to plan your care. They should also support your family, carers or other people who are important to you.

You have the right to express your wishes about where you would like to receive care and where you want to die. You can receive end of life care at home, or in care homes, hospices or hospitals, depending on your needs and preference.

People who are approaching the end of life are entitled to high-quality care, wherever they're being cared for.

Professionals who Provides End of Life Care

Different health and social care professionals may be involved in your end of life care, depending on your needs. For example, hospital doctors and nurses, your GP, community nurses, hospice staff and counsellors may all be involved, as well as social care staff, chaplains (of all faiths or none), physiotherapists, occupational therapists or complementary therapists.

If you are being cared for at home or in a care home, your GP has overall responsibility for your care. Community nurses usually visit you at home, and family and friends may be closely involved in caring for you too.

Palliative Care

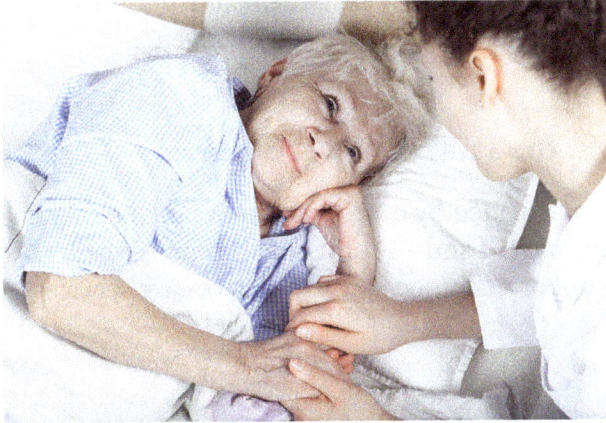

Palliative care is an approach that improves the quality of life of patients and their families facing the problem associated with life-threatening illness, through the prevention and relief of suffering by means of early identification and impeccable assessment and treatment of pain and other problems, physical, psychosocial and spiritual. Palliative care:

- Provides relief from pain and other distressing symptoms;

- Affirms life and regards dying as a normal process;

- Intends neither to hasten or postpone death;

- Integrates the psychological and spiritual aspects of patient care;

- Offers a support system to help patients live as actively as possible until death;

- Offers a support system to help the family cope during the patients illness and in their own bereavement;

- Uses a team approach to address the needs of patients and their families, including bereavement counselling, if indicated;

- Will enhance quality of life, and may also positively influence the course of illness;

- Is applicable early in the course of illness, in conjunction with other therapies that are intended to prolong life, such as chemotherapy or radiation therapy, and includes those investigations needed to better understand and manage distressing clinical complications.

Palliative care is for people of any age who have been told that they have a serious illness that cannot be cured. Palliative care assists people with illnesses such as cancer, motor neurone disease and end-stage kidney or lung disease to manage symptoms and improve quality of life.

For some people, palliative care may be beneficial from the time of diagnosis with a serious life-limiting illness. Palliative care can be given alongside treatments given by other doctors.

People who are in the Palliative Care Team

Palliative care may be provided by a wide range of people, this may include your GP, aged care worker, cardiologist and any other health care provider, as do family and other carers. They are supported by specialist palliative care services if symptoms become difficult to manage.

Places where Palliative Care is Provided

Palliative care is provided where the person and their family wants, where possible. This may include:

- At home

- In hospital

- In a hospice

- In a residential aged care facility.

Many people indicate a preference to die at home and making this possible often depends on several factors, including:

- The nature of the illness and amount of care the person needs

- How much support is available from the person's family and community

- Whether the person has someone at home who can provide physical care and support for them.

Hospice Care

Hospice care is the treatment given to prevent, control, or relieve complications and side effects and to improve the patient's comfort and quality of life.

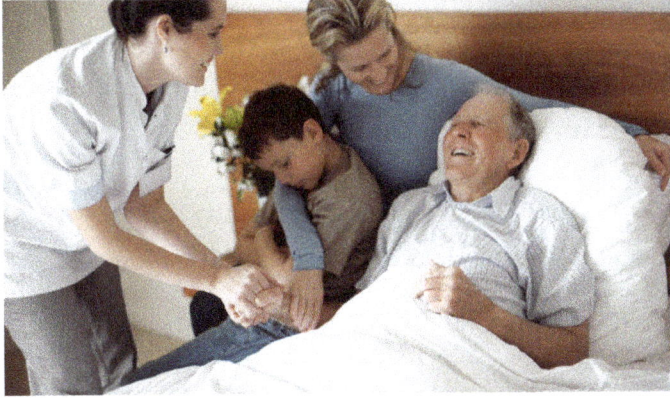

Hospice Facts

- Hospice care is a service, which may be provided at home, in a hospital, a nursing home, or in a facility specifically designated for such service.

- Hospice does not hasten or prolong death.

- Hospice care may be recommended for patients with a usually less than six-month life expectancy and an incurable illness for whom the focus of care is primarily comfort.

- The goal of hospice is to provide comfort, reduce suffering, and preserve patient dignity.

- A team consisting of doctors, nurses, social workers, clerics, volunteers, and therapists participate in the care of hospice patients.

- Medicare, Medicaid, and most private insurance carriers provide hospice benefits.

Hospice is a field of medicine that focuses on the comprehensive care of patients with terminal illnesses. Hospice need not be a place but rather a service that offers support, resources, and assistance to terminally ill patients and their families.

The main goal of hospice is to provide a peaceful, symptom-free, and dignified transition to death for patients whose diseases are advanced beyond a cure. The hope for a cure shifts to hope for a life free of suffering. The focus becomes quality of life rather than its length.

Hospice care is patient-centered medical care. A host of valuable services are offered to address every aspect of the patient's care as a whole. This is achieved by considering each individual's goals, values, beliefs, and rituals.

Importance of Hospice Care

In many chronic and progressive conditions such as cancer, heart disease, or dementia, the natural disease process can ultimately reach an end stage. Most of the time, as a disease progresses to an advanced stage, its symptoms become more intolerable and difficult to control. As a result, an end-stage condition can significantly impair a person's functional status and quality of life.

At this point, often there is no further cure or treatment to control the progression of the disease. Furthermore, aggressive treatment may only offer little benefit while posing significant risk and jeopardizing the patient's quality of life.

In such late stages of diseases, hospice can offer help for patients and families. The use of the term "nothing left to do," is generally to be avoided by health care professionals. There may be nothing with curative potential to do, but there is always something to do that helps with symptoms or improves quality of life. There are many aspects of a patient's well-being that can be addressed. Hospice can play a key role in managing physical symptoms of a disease (palliative care) and supporting patients and families emotionally and spiritually.

Hospice care promotes open discussions about "the big picture" with patients and their loved ones. The disease process, prognosis, and realities are often important parts of these discussions. More importantly, the patient's wishes, values, and beliefs are taken into account and become the cornerstone of the hospice plan of care.

Hospice and palliative care philosophy encourages these type of discussions with treating physicians early on in the course of a terminal disease. Patients can outline their preferences before they become too ill and incapable, thereby relieving some of the decision-making burden from family members. Advance care directives can be discussed and their completion facilitated in this setting.

Main Goals of Hospice Care

The end-of-life period is a sensitive part of everyone's life cycle. Psychosocial, financial, interpersonal, medical, and spiritual conflicts are all intertwined.

The main goal of hospice care is to reduce potentially unavoidable physical, emotional, psychosocial, and spiritual suffering encountered by patients during the dying process.

As a result, medical care during this period is very delicate and needs to be individually tailored. End-of-life care requires detailed attention to each person's wishes, beliefs, values, social situation, and personal characteristics.

The complex care of hospice patients may include the following:

- Managing evolving medical issues (infections, medication management, pressure ulcers, hydration, nutrition, physical stages of dying).

- Treating physical symptoms (pain, shortness of breath, anxiety, nausea, vomiting, constipation, confusion, etc.).

- Counseling about the anxiety, uncertainty, grief, and fear associated with end of life and dying.

- Rendering support to the patient, their families, and caregivers with the overwhelming physical and psychological stresses of a terminal illness.

- Guiding patients and families through the difficult interpersonal and psychosocial issues and helping them with finding closure.

- Paying attention to personal, religious, spiritual, and cultural values.

- Assisting patients and families making their wishes known and also reaching financial closures (living will, trust, advance directive, funeral arrangements).

- Providing bereavement counseling to the mourning loved ones after the death of the patient.

Misconceptions Regarding Hospice Care

Many misconceptions about hospice care still exist in the mind of the public and health care professionals. For example, it is perceived that hospice is a physical location and it only treats painin cancer patients.

The following are some of the true facts about hospice to clarify these misconceptions:

- Hospice care can be provided in many settings. It need not be only a physical place where patients go to die.

- Hospice is not only for cancer patients.

- Hospice does not deal only with pain management.

- Hospice does not hasten or prolong death.

- Hospice does not discriminate based on age, gender, race, or religion.

- Hospice does not participate in or encourage active euthanasia.

- Hospice does permit patients to see their regular physician.

- Hospice does allow patients to go to hospital if they choose.

- Hospice can be revoked at any time by patients or their families.

- Hospice can be provided for children with terminal disease.

Kinds of Services Hospice Care Provide

Services provided under hospice depend on the patient's needs and medical condition. General services provided by hospice include:

- Routine medical assessment and evaluation by a physician,

- Frequent nurse visits ranging between daily to weekly depending on patient's needs and condition,

- Spiritual counseling,

- Social worker evaluation,

- Volunteer services.

Additional personnel, including dieticians, pharmacists, home health aids, and other therapists, can also be involved in the care of a patient under hospice.

Contribution from these team members is dictated by the needs and goals of the patient.

In regards to medications, hospice typically supplies medications that help with managing and controlling the symptoms of the underlying condition.

In addition, durable medical equipment and medical supplies are routinely provided and covered under hospice benefits. Wheelchairs, hospital beds, wound care supplies, oxygen tanks, nutritional supplements, diapers, and urinary catheters are examples of some of the equipment often provided to patients by hospice.

Are Hospice Services Available for Children? Most, but not all, hospices render care for pediatric patients with terminal illnesses. The care provided for children on hospice is generally even more delicate and complex because of:

- Challenges in communicating with children about their illness,

- Children's perceptions about illness and death,

- Difficulty assessing children's symptoms,

- Unnatural and dramatic circumstance for parents,

- Effects of a child's illness on other siblings and friends,

- Uneasy social interactions with other children.

Hospices which provide pediatric care often use the expertise of counselors, therapists, and social workers trained in child psychology and communication.

Hospice Care Offered at Home

Yes, because hospice is a service which can be provided in many different settings. Its location to deliver care is based on each individual's preference. In fact, the majority of patients on hospice stay at their home or their usual residence (nursing homes or long-term care facilities) as they did prior to going on hospice.

Hospice care can be offered where the patient lives as long as the environment is safe, and the intensity of care does not overwhelm the patient and caregivers. Occasionally, a patient may need to be moved to a nursing facility or another health care setting if their home care becomes unachievable. This situation usually arises because of a need for higher level of personal care or uncontrolled symptoms requiring close monitoring by trained staff.

What are Some Medical Conditions Commonly Referred to Hospice?

Even though cancer remains one of the most common hospice diagnoses, many other terminal conditions are now very routinely referred to hospice.

Conditions other than cancer that are commonly referred to hospice are:

- Lung disease (chronic obstructive lung disease, COPD);
- Heart disease, congestive heart failure;
- Stroke;
- Coma;
- Advanced liver disease, cirrhosis;
- End-stage kidney disease;
- Dementia (Alzheimer's or other types);
- Advanced neurologic diseases (Parkinson's disease, ALS);
- Human immunodeficiency virus (HIV)/AIDS.

In reality, no specific restrictions exist as to what conditions can be referred to hospice. Any disease that is deemed end stage is not reversible, and its further treatment poses more burden than benefit can be considered for referral to hospice.

Hospice focuses on patients with terminal illnesses living out their last days in comfort. Hospice care is recommended for patients who have received diagnoses of less than 6 months to live due to terminal illnesses, such as cancer or Alzheimer's. Hospice is family-oriented, as the family stays involved in all aspects of decision-making and patient care, while a team of hospice caregivers attend to patient monitoring, medications, and therapy. If you or a loved one is facing a terminal illness, use these tips to learn how to arrange hospice care.

Determining Eligibility

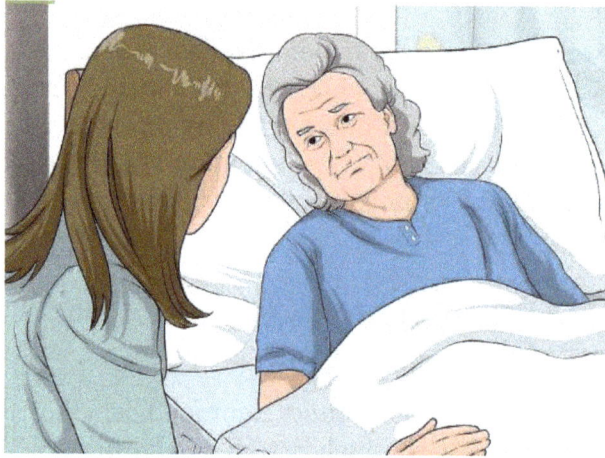

1. Watch for signs it may be time to move to hospice: A number of signs can point to the fact that it may be time for the patient to enter hospice care. For instance, the patient may stay in bed all the time, contract more infections, have more pain, and experience rapid weight loss. The patient may also be increasingly weaker, as well as needing to visit the hospital more often. In addition, you may notice signs that your loved one is getting worse, despite still taking drugs to cure the disease.

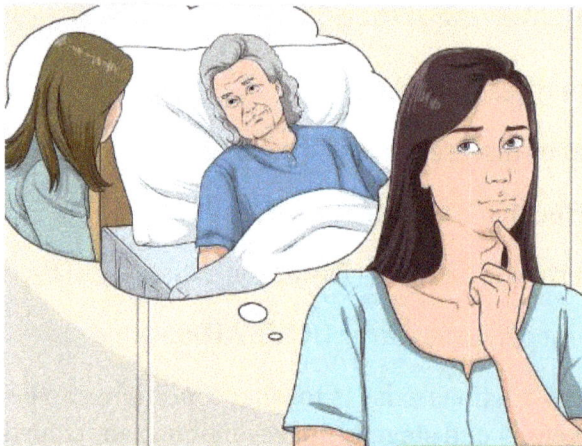

2. Make sure the patient is ready for hospice care: Hospice is intended to make the patient's life more comfortable as they deal with a terminal illness. It's not intended to treat the disease the patient has, except for pain management. In other words, if the patient still wants to fight the disease through treatments like chemotherapy or a transplant, it's not time for hospice yet.

- Keep in mind that hospice care doesn't provide interventions that prolong life, such as feeding tubes, unless the patient already has a feeding tube before entering hospice care.

- It can be difficult to have this conversation. You have to open it up with sensitivity and care. It can also be helpful for you to involve health care providers because they have lots of experience having this conversation. Plus, they know all about the benefits of hospice.

- If you choose to have the conversation alone, start by saying what kind of care hospice offers. You could say, "We may need to start thinking about hospice. Hospice covers pain management, medication coordination, and daily care. Just because you accept hospice doesn't mean you can't go back to treatment later."

- You might also mention that Hospice workers are kind, caring, and experienced in all aspects.

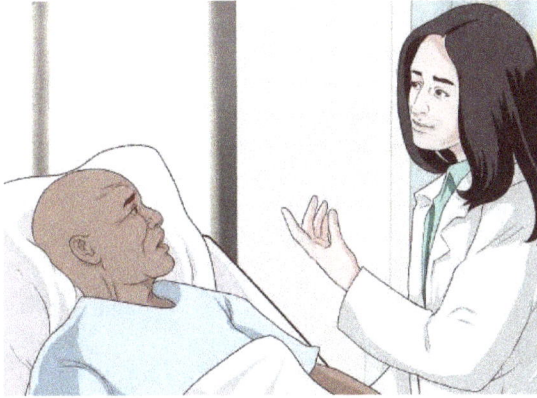

3. Have a doctor certify the patient for hospice care: To be in hospice care, particularly if the care needs to be covered by Medicare, the patient needs to be certified by a doctor. Generally, that means that the patient has a terminal illness and can't be reasonably expected to live more than 6 months.

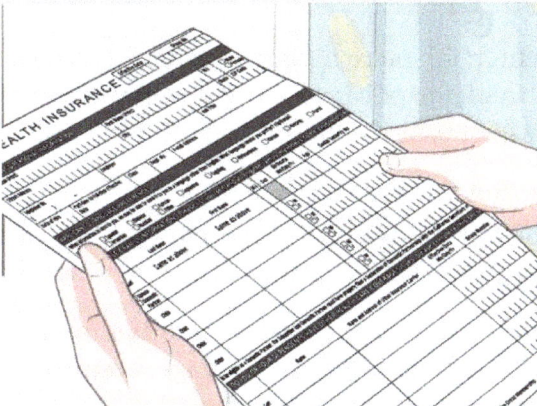

4. Understand how payment works: You don't want to be worrying about money as someone's life draws to a close, but often, money can become an issue. Luckily, hospice is covered in full by Medicare, and it's also covered in part or in full by many major insurance companies.

- However, if you aren't covered by Medicaid, Medicare, veteran's insurance like tricare, or private insurance usually cover hospice care. However, you may need to pay for hospice out of pocket if it is not covered. Many nonprofits will provide some relief for people who must pay out of pocket, such as paying on a sliding scale.

- Though hospice is cheaper than hospital care, it can still be expensive, running as much as $600 or more per day, though it can be as little as $150 per day, depending on what services the patient is receiving. This amount is usually subsidized (partially covered) by your insurance company. However, you should still check with your provider to see what you might owe out-of-pocket.

Contacting a Hospice Center

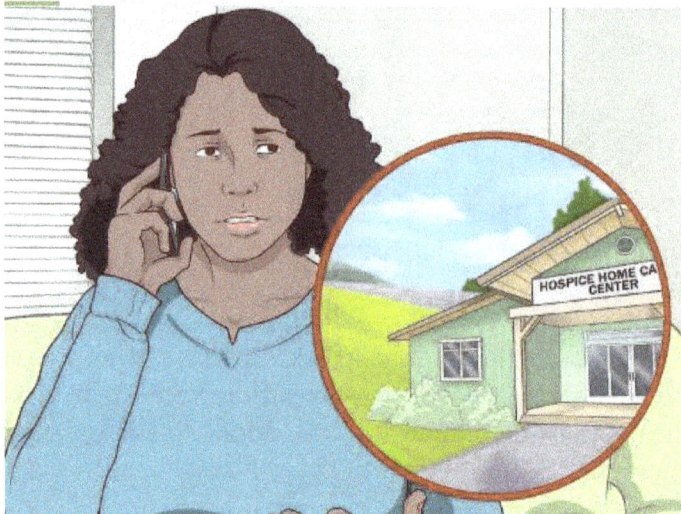

1. Contact a hospice center: If you're a family member, you can initiate contact with hospice. The patient or their doctor can also begin contact. With the initial contact, you will just be discussing what hospice entails. You're not committing to it yet.

- Usually, your doctor will recommend a hospice center. Generally, a nonprofit hospice is recommended. However, you can call any hospice center in your area that you feel is appropriate for you.

- You can also find local hospices through organizations like the American Cancer Society, United Way, or the Agency on Aging. These organizations often provide referrals to local hospices.

- Another way to pick a hospice is to ask friends and family for recommendations. Many people have been in the same place you have, and they can offer guidance about the agencies in town.

- Often, a hospice nurse will come to the hospital, house, or nursing home where the patient is staying at the time to discuss hospice care.

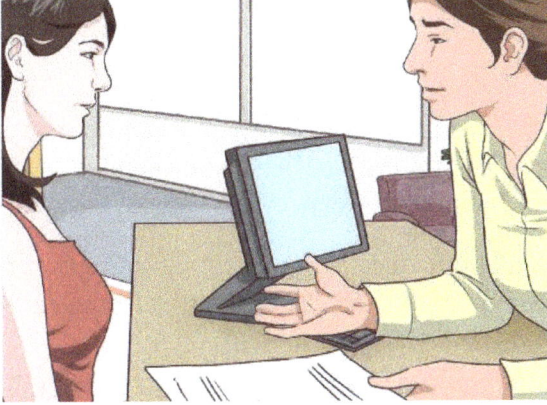

2. Verify that your agency has the proper certifications: Your agency should be accredited through a national agency, such as the Joint Commission. In addition, it should be Medicare-approved, since that approval requires that the agency meet certain standards. Some states also require that the agency be licensed, which you can look up through your state.

- When meeting with the agency, you can ask about their accreditation, certification, and licensing, or you can look the information up online.

- Don't be afraid to go to another agency if you're not comfortable with what one is telling you. It is fine to shop around with other agencies to see what they offer, but keep in mind that all of the nurses will be through hospice.

- The Joint Commission is a national accrediting agency that provides accreditation for approximately 21,000 health organizations in the United States.

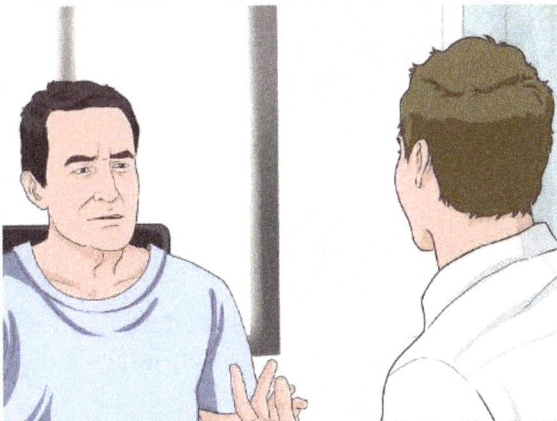

3. Ask questions: When you visit with the hospice worker, feel free to ask questions. That's why they are there. They want you and the patient to feel comfortable with the decision to go with hospice, so don't be afraid to put your fears out there. The hospice worker understands, and they are trained to be compassionate and caring.

- Ask about things like how soon care can be started (right away is best), what requirements the agency has for in-patient care, whether the patient can continue on certain treatments (such as dialysis), and exactly what kinds of care hospice provides for the patient.

- Also ask if the caregivers are on-call anytime (24 hours a day) and whether they personalize care plans for each patient. You can also ask about who will be providing care and what you'll be expected to do.

- If you don't get all your questions answered in the first meeting, you'll have a chance to talk again. Most hospice centers welcome calls, and many will send someone out to meet with you more than once.

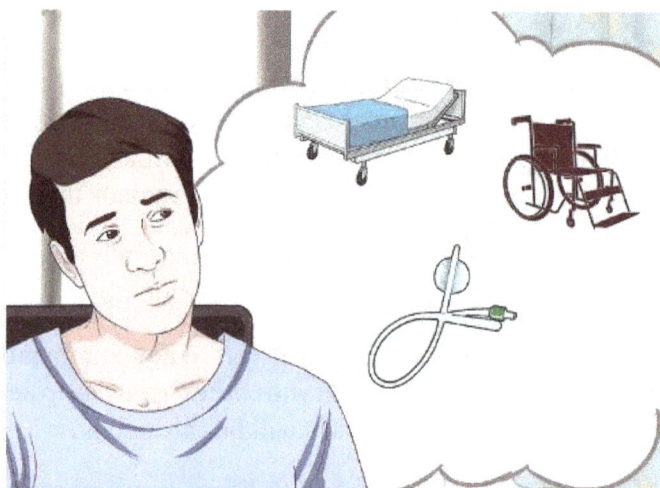

4. Learn what hospice covers: Hospice covers everything from care to equipment. They can provide nursing and doctor care. They can also provide equipment, such as hospital beds, wheelchairs, walkers, and bedside toilets, as well as supplies, such as catheters, bed pans, bed pads, and gloves. The patient will also be given medications appropriate for palliative care, such as pain medications, and will also be provided with nursing aid care, such as showering or bathing several times a week.

- Other services may include diabetes counseling, physical therapy, spiritual guidance (from a chaplain), and nutritional advice.

- For the family, hospice can provide short-term and long-term respite care, meaning hospice can care for the patient 24-hours a day for a period (usually up to 5 days) if the primary caregiver needs a break.

- Keep in mind that hospice covers in home care and hospital care as needed. A hospice nurse will visit the patient at home, and the nurse may also recommend that the patience be admitted to the hospital.

- Hospice does not cover medications intended to cure the disease rather than manage pain.

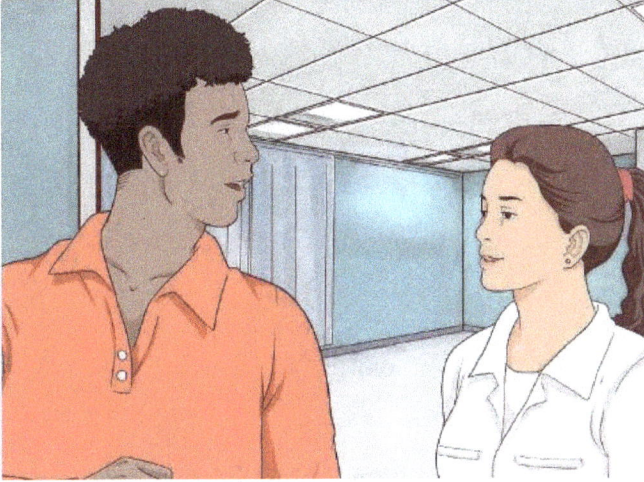

5. Don't be afraid to say "yes": Hospice sounds scary because it may seem like you're giving up on the person's care. However, if the person has a terminal illness, hospice can provide care to make the person more comfortable, meaning the end of the person's life will be better. Plus, hospice can provide a wide variety of care that helps relieve you and other people in charge of the person's care, so that you can focus on being with the person rather than caring for the person.

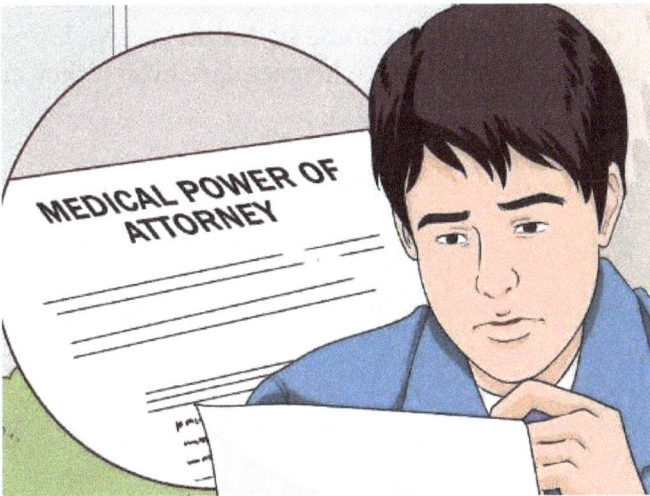

6. Make the decision, if you need to do so: If you're the person's medical power of attorney, it may fall to you to make the decision for hospice. Often in the final days of an

illness, the person becomes confused and unable to make informed decisions, which is why they named a person they trusted to make the decision for them (you, possibly). In that case, you may need to decide that the person needs to enter hospice care, and legally, you have the right to do so.

Opening the Door to Hospice Care

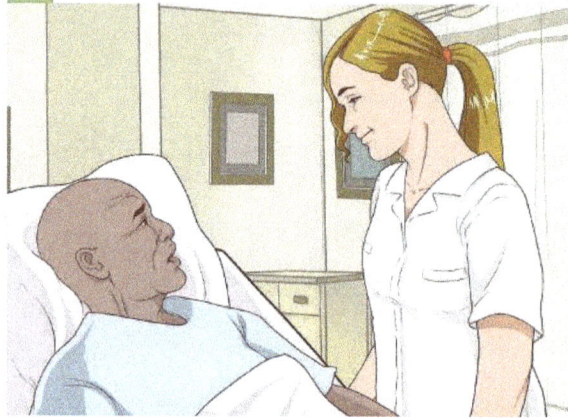

1. Be ready for hospice to enter the home: Most hospice care is done in the patient's home or nursing home. Therefore, you need to be ready to have people in the patient's home at all hours of the day, though most care will be provided during the day. While in some cases, the patient may be moved to an in-patient hospice center, one of the benefits of hospice care is it can be done in the comfort of the patient's own home.

- Basically, all you need to get ready is to make space available for what hospice will bring in, such as a hospital bed.

- The patient doesn't need to be home-bound to receive hospice care. In other words, the patient can still receive hospice care even if they are still able to get out and about.

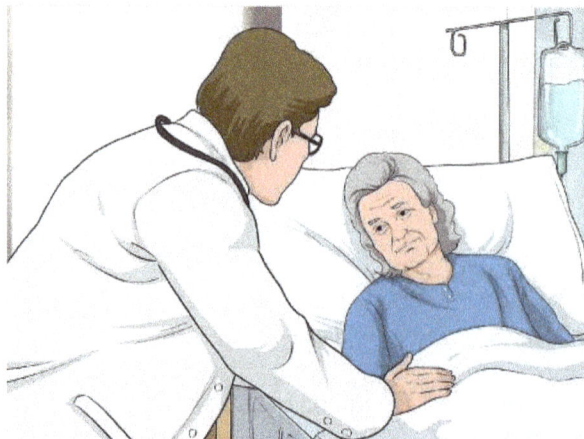

2. Continue seeing the patient's doctor: Most of the time, the doctor that is already caring for the patient becomes part of the hospice team. Therefore, you don't need to worry about switching to a new doctor at this difficult time. The patient will be able to have someone they know and trust on the team.

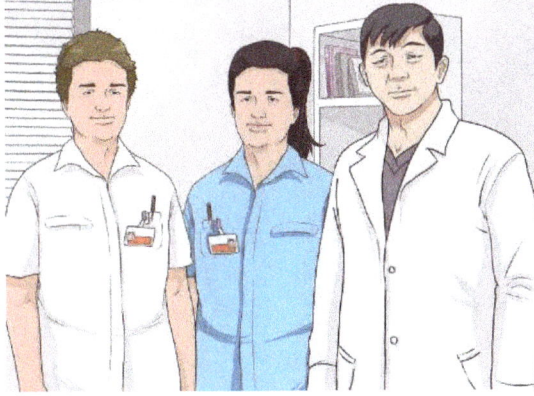

3. Let hospice coordinate care: One of the benefits of having hospice care is that they will coordinate the patient's care. In other words, they will give information to the parties that need it, including the pharmacy and the patient's doctor, so you don't have to. You can focus on being with the person.

- The hospice team will be composed of many members, which can include a registered nurse, doctors, nursing aids, therapists, nutritionists, social workers, and trained volunteers, all ready to help provide care to your loved one.

- When the time does come, the team will also assist with connecting you to the funeral home of your choice, and they can do so at any time to help you make arrangements.

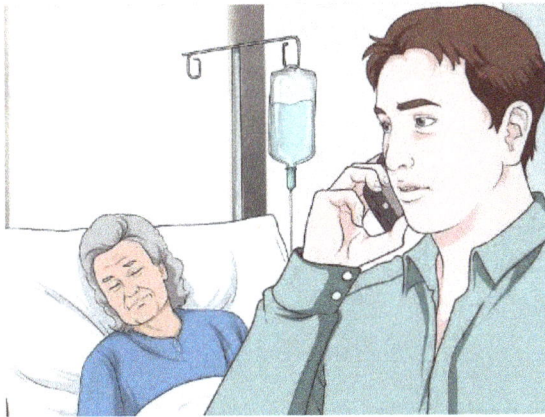

4. Don't be afraid to call: Hospice is meant to be there for you when you need it, even in the middle of the night. If something is happening with the patient, call hospice for help. They can either reassure you or send someone out to check on the patient.

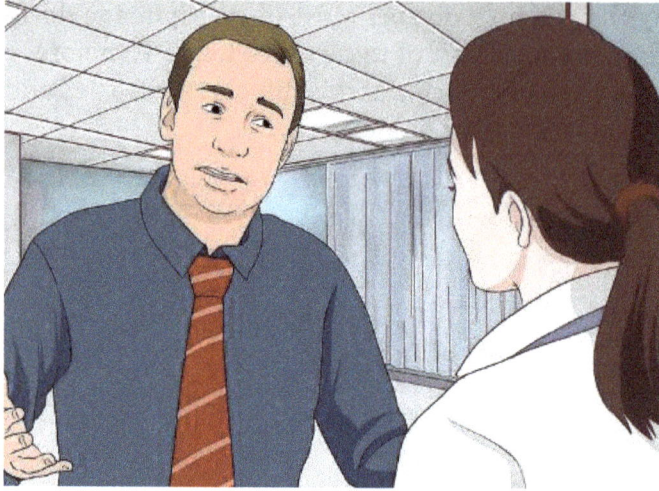

5. Prepare for the fact that the patient won't return to the hospital: While it is a benefit for the patient to be in their own homes, generally the patient will not return to hospital for any care. You will find hospice will make exceptions for injuries not related to the illness, such as the patient falling and cutting themselves, where stitches are required. However, the patient usually doesn't return to the hospital for care related to the terminal illness, though it does depend on the patient and the hospice program.

- When the patient needs to go to the hospital for something non-illness related, you usually need to inform hospice of what is happening.

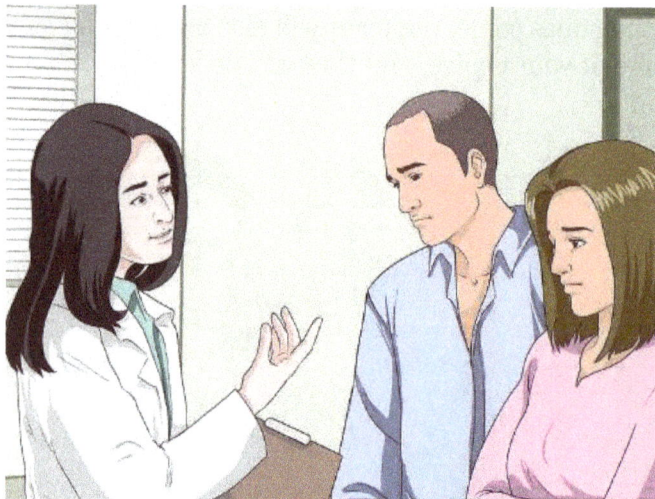

6. Accept the help that hospice offers the family: Hospice care of course provides relief for friends and family member by assisting with care. However, hospice also provides other services for friends and family, such as having regular meetings to keep family updated, as well as bereavement care when the patient finally passes.

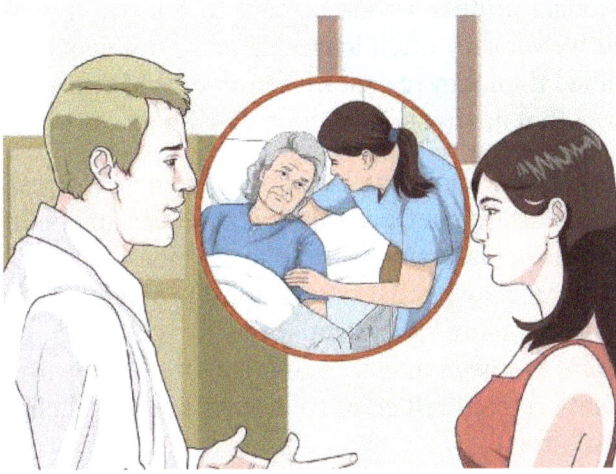

7. End hospice care if you feel it's appropriate: Once you commit to hospice care, you and the patient are saying that you just want palliative care, not curative care, meaning you're not looking to cure the patient's disease. However, you can stop hospice care at any point if the patient or a family member decides that they want to pursue cures again. Therefore, you are able to change your mind if new information comes to light.

- However, the person cannot be pushed off hospice by the provider or by Medicare. Once the person is in hospice, they'll remain, even if they live beyond the "6 months" certified by the doctor.

Spiritual Care

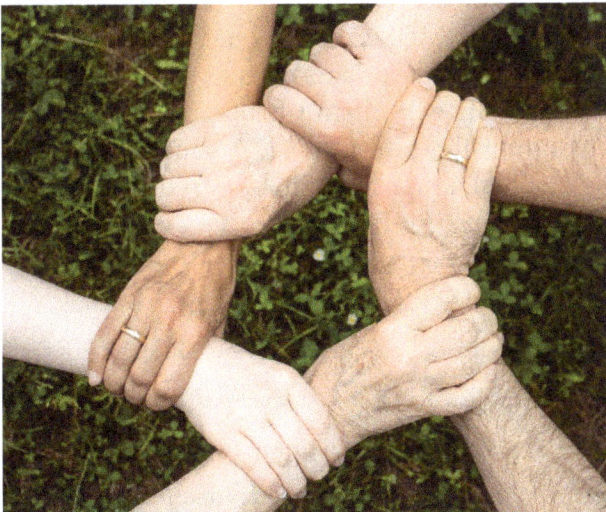

Spiritual care is that aspect of health care that attends to spiritual and religious needs brought on by an illness or injury

Health care professionals profess a commitment to holistic care, in which the whole person is ministered to, yet they often leavespiritual problems to persons whom they consider better qualified than they to deal with problems of this kind. Thus patient soften have deep concerns that are unspoken and suffering that is not shared.

Assessment of spiritual needs should go beyond a perfunctory question about religious affiliation at the time of admission. Questions about values and beliefs should be asked, preferably at the end of the assessment interview, when the patient shows trust and confidence in the nurse. It may be that patients will provide little information at first, but later on, when thereis a more trusting relationship with the nurse, or when a frightening medical diagnosis has been made, assessment andinter ventions may be indicated. However, if patients remain reluctant to discuss personal beliefs and values, their right to privacy is respected.

Stoll has suggested that there are four general areas of concern to be addressed during spiritual assessment. These include (1) the person's concept of God or deity and how this concept is significant in his or her life; (2) sources of help and strength in times of spiritual crises; (3) religious practices; and (4) the relation between spiritual beliefs and health, sickness, and death.

Profound questions of the meaning of suffering and death may surface when a person is experiencing a serious illness or similar crisis of physical health. In the face of impending death or a radical change imposed by the loss of a body part or function, patients may experience panic, anxiety, depression, and feelings of guilt or abandonment. They need opportunities to express spiritual concerns to an attentive listener, to bring into focus and work through their questions and doubts, and to experience hope and support for the beliefs that give them strength and consolation.

While health care providers are not typically the primary source of spiritual counsel, they can contribute to the overallwelfare of their patients by being alert for expressions of spiritual distress, listening to the patients when they want to talkabout spiritual concerns, and reading and praying with them when appropriate. Referral to the hospital chaplain or thepatient's minister, priest, or other spiritual guide is an important part of meeting a patient's spiritual needs, but it does notrelieve health care professionals of their responsibility for continued spiritual support.

References

- What-it-involves-and-when-it-starts, end-of-life-care: nhs.uk, Retrieved 11 July 2018

- What-is-palliative-care: palliativecare.org.au, Retrieved 08 April 2018

- What-is-hospice-care: medicinenet.com, Retrieved 29 June 2018

- Arrange-Hospice-Care: wikihow.com, Retrieved 11 June 2018

- Spiritual-care: medical-dictionary.thefreedictionary.com, Retrieved 28 May 2018

Specimen Collection

Specimen collection, handling and preparation are important tasks performed by a nurse. Gathering samples in a way that ensures self-protection and prevents the spread of diseases is part of a nurse's core responsibilities. The topics elaborated in this chapter address the role of nurses in specimen collection, its techniques of handling, etc.

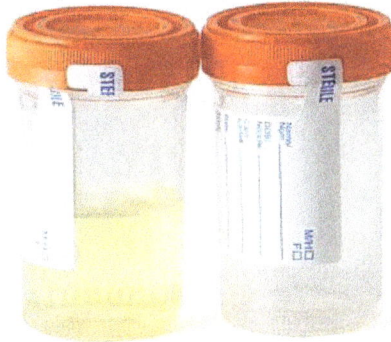

Specimen collection, preparation and handling are important tasks performed by nurses. By identifying pathogens and analyzing urine, feces, sputum and blood, one can assess the health status of a patient. One of the core responsibilities of nurses is to collect, then label specimens for analysis. Immediately after this, the specimens should be delivered to the lab.

Nurses need to be aware of how to properly gather specimens, both for self-protection, and to prevent the spread of diseases.

Principles of Specimen Collection

If possible, collect the specimen in the acute phase of the infection and before antibiotics are administered.

- Select the correct anatomic site for collection of the specimen.

- Collect the specimen using the proper technique and supplies with minimal contamination from normal biota (normal flora).

- Collect the appropriate quantity of specimen.

- Package the specimen in a container designed to maintain the viability of the organisms.

- Label the specimen accurately with the specific anatomic site and the patient informations.

- Transport the specimen to the laboratory promptly.

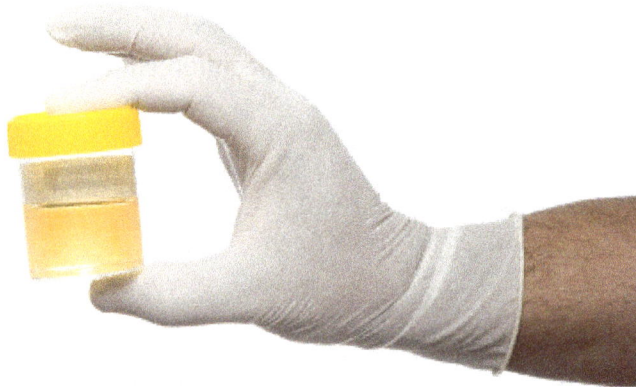

Specimen Collection Guidelines

Blood Culture: Disinfect skin with alcohol and iodine, blood culture media set (aerobic and anaerobic, bottles) or vacutainer tube with SPS(sodium polyanethol sulfonate) / adults, 20 ml per set; children 5 to 10 ml per set.

Body Fluids: (Abdominal, amniotic, ascites, bile, joint, pericardial, pleural), disinfect skin before needle aspiration sterile, screw-cap tube ≥ 1 ml.

Cerebrospinal Fluid: Disinfect skin before aspiration, use sterile screw-cap tube/bacteria ≥ 1 ml, fungi, ≥ 2 ml, AFB ≥ 2 ml, virus ≥ 1 ml.

Ear

1. Inner ear: clean ear canal with mild soap, aspirate fluid, with needle if eardrum intact; Or use swab if , eardrum ruptured, sterile, screw-cap tube or anaerobic transport system.

2. Outer ear : remove debris or crust from ear canal with saline moistened swab; rotate swab in outer canal, swab transport system.

Feces Samples

- Collect directly into container, avoid contamination with urine, clean, leakproof container or enteric transport system.

- A rectal swab can be submitted for bacterial culture but it must show feces. A single specimen is not usually sufficient to exclude bacteria or parasites.

- if a bacterial infection is suspected, three specimens should be collected, one a day for 3 days.

- if parasites are suspected, three specimens collected within 10 days should be sufficient for microscopic detection of ova and parasites.

- The newer methods detect parasite antigens, and one sample is usually sufficient.

- Commercial systems are available with preservatives for bacteria and parasites. The appropriate ratio of stool to preservative is 1:3

Fungal Scrapings

Wipe nails or skin with alcohol , use clean, screw-cap container.

- Hair/nails/skin hair: 10-12 hairs with shaft intact

- Nails: clip affected area

- Skin: scrape skin at outer edge of lesion.

Genitalia

- Cervix/Vagina : Remove mucus before collection; do not use lubricant on speculum; swab endocervical canal or vaginal mucosa, swab transport system or JEMBEC transport system.

- Urethra : Flexible swab inserted 2-4 cm into urethra for 2-3 sec or collect discharge, swab transport system or JEMBEC transport system.

- Lesion/Wound/Abscess: Wipe area with sterile saline or alcohol , superficial swab along outer edge, swab transport system, deep aspirate with needle and syringe, anaerobic transport system.

Respiratory Tract: Lower Bronchial Specimens

- Sputum, Rinse Mouth Or Gargle With Water, Instruct To Cough Deeply Into Container. Or the patient should rinse the mouth with water and expectorate with the aid of a deep cough directly into a sterile container (expectorated sputum).

- Patients with dentures should remove the dentures first. A single specimen should be adequate for detection of bacterial LRT infection. If fungal or mycobacterial infections are possible, three separate early morning specimens (collected on successive days) are appropriate.

- Specimens may be collected through aerosol-induction in which the patient breathes aerosolized droplets of a solution that stimulates cough reflex (induced sputum).

Respiratory Tract: URT

1. Nasal : Insert premoistened swab with sterile saline 1 inch into nares, swab , use transport system.

2. Nasopharynx : Insert flexible swab through nose into posterior nasopharynx, rotate for 5 sec, swab transport system or direct inoculation to media.

3. Throat Swab, Posterior pharynx, tonsils, and inflamed areas, swab transport system.

Role of Nurses in Specimen Collection

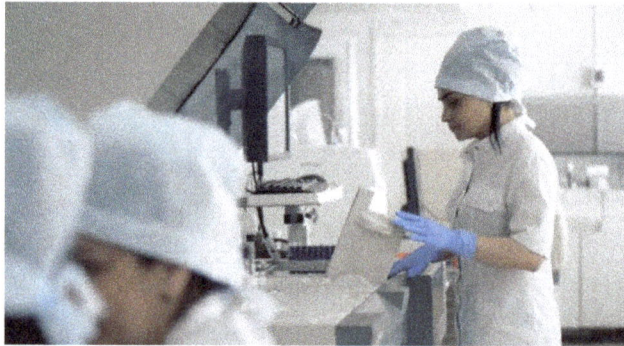

- Ensuring appropriate collection of samples.

- Precise sample identification.

- Making sure all selected supplies are suitable for collection.

- Timely transfer of specimen to the lab.

- Patient interaction.

Common Specimen Collections

Throat Swab Culture

To check the presence of a bacterial or fungal infection in the throat, a diagnostic test called a throat swab culture is conducted. In this test, a sample of mucus is collected on a cotton-tipped applicator and is placed on a special cup that allows infections to dwell. Common infections include pneumonia, whooping cough, and tonsillitis.

Sputum Specimen and Culture

In this laboratory analysis, a sample of material is expelled from the respiratory passages to determine pathogen presence. It generally takes a good 2-3 days to collect the specimen, as it is very difficult for a patient to cough up enough sputum at one time.

Stool Specimen and Culture

Stool cultures include the process of growing organisms existing in the feces to identify any disease-causing bacteria. The most common is the parasites and ova test to detect the presence of parasites such as amoebas or worms.

Urine Specimen and Culture

Physical, chemical and microscopic examination of urine is referred to as urinalysis. It generally involves a number of tests to analyze various compounds thoroughly that pass through the urine. The color, density, and odor of the urine are all considered to reveal the individual's health status.

Caring for Physical Injuries or Wounds

The first stage in the treatment of any wound or a physical injury is in the evaluation of the cause, type and depth of the wound. The treatment involves cleaning, closing and dressing the wound. The management of wounds is an area of nursing care. This chapter explores the diverse aspects of wounds, wound care, wound first aid and wound care dressing.

Wounds

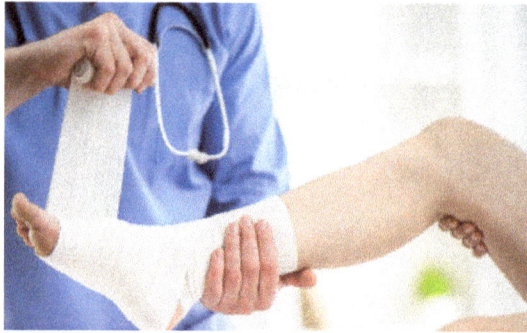

Wound is a break in the continuity of any bodily tissue due to violence, where violence is understood to encompass any action of external agency, including, for example, surgery. Within this general definition many subdivisions are possible, taking into account and grouping together the various forms of violence or tissue damage.

The most important distinction is between open and closed wounds. Open wounds are those in which the protective body surface (the skin or mucous membranes) has been broken, permitting the entry of foreign material into the tissues. In closed wounds, by contrast, the damaged tissues are not exposed to the exterior, and the process of repair can take place without the interference that contamination brings, in greater or lesser degree. Further divisions may be made on the basis of the mode of production of the wound.

Closed Wounds

The degree of injury sustained from a direct blow depends upon the force of the blow and its direction. Obviously the degree of damage increases with increasing force. The effects of direction are equally important, although not so readily appreciated.

For example, a hammer blow to the side of the head may severely bruise the scalp or, delivered with equal force but directed in a slightly different way, may cause extensive damage to the base of the skull. Anatomic and physiologic factors may also affect the degree of injury. Thus, a fall on an outstretched hand may have extremely different effects on a child, a young adult, and an elderly person.

A relatively slight blow may damage the skin and underlying soft tissues, as shown by bruising, or contusion, which results from the infiltration of blood into the tissues from ruptured small vessels and by swelling caused by the passage of fluid through the walls of damaged capillaries. As a rule, the hemorrhage ceases abruptly, the blood and fluid are absorbed within a few days, and the part is restored to normal. When larger vessels are injured, much more blood escapes, and it collects in the tissues and forms a mass called a hematoma.

A direct, forceful blow may damage any of the underlying tissues; blood vessels, nerves, muscles, bones, joints, or the internal organs may be affected. Damage to the deeper tissues may result from the direct impact of the blow upon a tissue, as in the fracturing of a skull by a hammer or, more commonly, from the transmission of the force of impact through the body to a relatively weak point. Thus, a fall on an outstretched hand may injure the flesh and bones of the hand itself, but a common result is a break at some other site in the arm through which the force is transmitted—at the scaphoid bone in the wrist, at the radius in the forearm just above the wrist, at the elbow, or at the shoulder—the breaking point being determined by the direction of force and the anatomy of the individual.

Other common forms of indirect injury result from twisting, as occurs when a person's foot becomes caught and he or she twists upon it, suffering, if the force is great enough, a sprained or broken ankle or a broken leg or hip; from bending; or from deceleration, a form of injury frequently encountered in automobile and aircraft accidents, where one part of the body is fixed while another is relatively mobile, giving rise, in abrupt stops, to a displacement of the mobile parts, commonly called whiplash.

Open Wounds

When the skin—or, in the case of injuries of the base of the skull or the sinuses, the mucous membrane—is broken, a wound is exposed to additional hazards, since the tissues may be invaded by foreign material such as bacteria, dirt, and fragments of clothing, which may give rise to serious local or general complications from infection. Furthermore, if the break in the skin is large, the resulting exposure of the wounded tissues to the drying and cooling effects of the air may increase the damage caused by the wounding agent itself.

A needle or a sharp knife that passes through the tissues with ease, dividing them cleanly or separating them, will produce relatively little damage except to those tissues directly in its course, and, indeed, unless an important structure is injured, the wounds caused are seldom serious. On the other hand, a bomb fragment, irregular and jagged, will, as it churns and rips through the soft tissues, produce extensive damage for a considerable distance in all directions. Likewise, the injury caused by crushing is frequently serious.

Skin, being sturdy and elastic and well supplied with blood, tolerates injury well and recovers quickly. The subcutaneous fatty tissues are more delicate and more easily deprived of their blood supply. Muscle, likewise, is sensitive to the damaging effect of shrapnel, being readily torn and unable to survive diminished blood supply for any appreciable time. Muscle, when damaged, is particularly prone to infection.

An injury to bone in an open wound is always serious, for any broken fragment detached from its blood supply will not survive if infection occurs, and it will remain as a foreign body in the wound to cause further complications. Even if the bone is cleanly broken and there are no loose fragments, infection may enter the raw surfaces of the fracture with disastrous results.

Clearly the seriousness of a wound is greatly increased if there is injury to a joint, a nerve, a major blood vessel, or an internal organ.

Contamination of a wound may occur at the moment of wounding or at any time thereafter until healing is complete. The effects of various nonbacterial contaminants vary considerably. In general, the critical factor for nonbacterial contaminants is the extent of the contamination. In the case of bacterial contaminants, the type of contaminant is of greater importance. Infection caused by virulent bacteria nourished by dead tissue and organic foreign material in the wound may take several forms, of which the three most important are: gas gangrene, the most dreaded, arising almost exclusively in damaged muscle tissue and spreading with alarming rapidity to cause death if unchecked by surgical or medical treatment; infections caused by organisms such as *Streptococcus* and *Staphylococcus* and the coliform bacteria, in which the local production of pus is a prominent feature accompanying a general reaction that may be severe; and tetanus, an often fatal infection that becomes evident some days after the wound has occurred, frequently without any marked local manifestations but characterized by generalized muscle spasms.

The final healing of a wound is the result of a series of complex biological events taking place over a long period. Viewed in the simplest way, in an untreated but uncomplicated wound, as from a clean knife cut, the process is as follows: When tissues are cut, the edges of the wound separate, apparently pulled apart by the elasticity of the skin. Blood from the severed blood vessel fills the cavity of the wound and overflows its edges. The blood clots and eventually the surface of the clot dries out and becomes hard, forming a scab. During the first 24 hours the scab shrinks, drawing the edges of the wound closer together. If the scab sloughs off or is removed after about a week, a layer of reddish granulation tissue will be seen to have covered the cut edges of the subcutaneous tissue. Gradually a pearly, grayish, thin membrane extends out from the skin edge; eventually it covers the whole surface. The actual area of the wound, meanwhile, is steadily reduced by a process of contraction; finally, there is no raw surface to be seen.

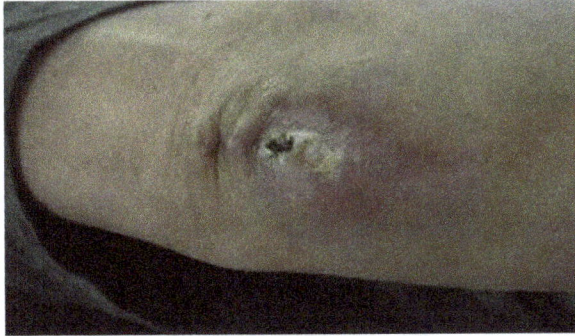

Wound

The thin linear scar that forms is at first red and raised above the level of the surrounding skin but gradually fades until it is considerably paler than the surrounding skin. For many weeks after the scar forms, this process of contracture continues as is shown by the gradual shortening of the wound. Wounds that cross normal "skin lines" tend, after several months, to widen and become depressed below the level of the surrounding skin. Scars do not tan in sunlight, and they produce neither hair nor sweat, all evidences of the failure of the skin to return to full function.

Microscopically one can observe in the clot the whole process of the development of fibrin that causes the clot to contract, the arrival of the white blood cells and the macrophages that digest the debris in the wound, and the growth of blood capillaries followed by the growth inward of fibrous tissue migrating from the cells on the margin of the wound. The fibres arising from these cells can be identified and seen to increase, eventually filling the wound cavity with a network of interlacing threads of the protein collagen that, influenced by lines of tension, finally range themselves in firm bands. Meanwhile, the surface of the wound is being covered by a process of enlargement and flattening and by multiplication of the preexisting skin cells at the edge of the wound. These covering, or epithelial, cells start very early to spread down into the wound, clearing a way for themselves beneath the scab, perhaps by the production of an enzyme that dissolves the deeper layers of the crust. Eventually the proliferating epithelial sheets from the two sides of the wound coalesce to heal the wound superficially.

Presentation

Complications

Bacterial infection of wound can impede the healing process and lead to life-threatening complications. Scientists at Sheffield University have used light to rapidly detect the presence of bacteria, by developing a portable kit in which specially designed molecules emit a light signal when bound to bacteria. Current laboratory-based detection of bacteria can take hours or days.

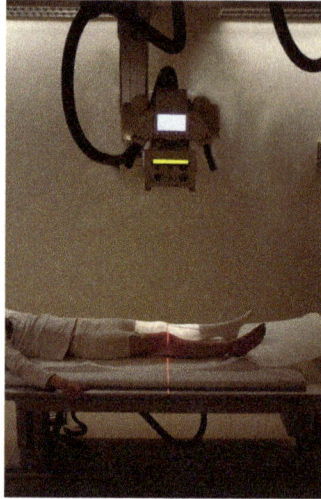

The patient has a deep wound at the knee, and radiography is used to
ensure there are no hidden bone fractures

Workup

Wounds that are not healing should be investigated to find the causes; many microbiological agents may be responsible. The basic workup includes evaluating the wound, its extent and severity. Cultures are usually obtained both from the wound site and blood. X-rays are obtained and a tetanus shot may be administered if there is any doubt about prior vaccination.

Chronic

Non-healing wounds of the diabetic foot are considered one of the most significant complications of diabetes, representing a major worldwide medical, social, and economic burden that greatly affects patient quality of life. Almost 24 million Americans—one in every twelve—are diabetic and the disease is causing widespread disability and death at an epidemic pace, according to the Centers for Disease Control and Prevention. Of those with diabetes, 6.5 million are estimated to suffer with chronic or non-healing wounds. Associated with inadequate circulation, poorly functioning veins, and immobility, non-healing wounds occur most frequently in the elderly and in people with diabetes—populations that are sharply rising as the nation ages and chronic diseases increase.

Although diabetes can ravage the body in many ways, non-healing ulcers on the feet and lower legs are common outward manifestations of the disease. Also, diabetics often suffer from nerve damage in their feet and legs, allowing small wounds or irritations to develop without awareness. Given the abnormalities of the microvasculature and other side effects of diabetes, these wounds take a long time to heal and require a specialized treatment approach for proper healing.

As many as 25% of diabetic patients will eventually develop foot ulcers, and recurrence within five years is 70%. If not aggressively treated, these wounds can lead to amputations. It is estimated that every 30 seconds a lower limb is amputated somewhere in the world because of a diabetic wound. Amputation often triggers a downward spiral of declining quality of life, frequently leading to disability and death. In fact, only about one third of diabetic amputees will live more than five years, a survival rate equivalent to that of many cancers.

Many of these lower extremity amputations can be prevented through an interdisciplinary approach to treatment involving a variety of advanced therapies and techniques, such as debridement, hyperbaric oxygen treatment therapy, dressing selection, special shoes, and patient education. When wounds persist, a specialized approach is required for healing.

Wound Care

Wound care refers to specific types of treatment for pressure sores , skin ulcers and other wounds that break the skin. Pressure ulcers, also called "bed sores" and referred to medically as decubitus ulcers, are wounds that commonly develop at pressure points on the body when the weight of an immobilized individual rests continuously on a hard surface such as a mattress or wheel chair. Uninterrupted pressure is the cause of pressure sores and relieving pressure is the mainstay of wound care. Other wounds that may benefit from specialized wound care techniques are diabetic foot ulcers, traumatic ulcers caused by injury, arterial and vein ulcers caused by lack of circulation, and burns.

Purpose

The purpose of wound care is twofold: 1) to relieve pressure on a weight-bearing part of the body such as a boney prominence (hand, arm, knee, heel, hip or buttocks) that rests on a bed, wheelchair, another body part, a splint or other hard object, and 2) to treat the ulcerated wound itself when skin has become weakened, inflamed and possibly infected. Although the current discussion of wound care relates primarily to pressure ulcers, other skin ulcers and burn wounds may benefit from similar treatment principles and practices.

Pressure sores develop in immobilized individuals who are constantly positioned the same way in a bed, chair or wheelchair or who may be in traction or paralyzed with limited range of motion. Older individuals who are compromised through acute or chronic illness, under heavy sedation or unconscious, or who have reduced mental functioning, typically do not receive normal nerve signals to move as mobile individuals do. Tissue damage may begin as tender inflamed areas over weight-bearing parts of the body that are in contact with a supporting surface such as a bed or wheelchair, or with another body part or a supportive device. Constant contact at these points exerts pressure on the skin and soft tissue, cutting off the normal flow of blood, oxygen and nutrients to tissue (ischemia), resulting in death of tissue cells (anoxia) and formation of pressure sores. The presence of sores is complicated by rubbing (shear) or friction between the supportive surface and skin over boney prominences. In compromised, immobilized individuals, skin breakdown can happen quickly within hours or days. Regular movement or turning of the individual is needed to relieve pressure, and clinical treatment of pressure sores is required to prevent infection and further breakdown.

Precautions

Physicians orders are required for wound care designed to prevent and treat pressure sores. Alertness to skin condition in immobilized patients is critical among caretakers and medical personal. Individuals at risk for pressure sores may only be aware of discomfort at the points of pressure and may not be aware of the presence of sores or the risk of infection. Caretakers should be informed of pressure sore risk and instructed about typical signs and preventive measures to protect the skin of at-risk individuals in their care.

Steps of Recovery

Wound care is usually ordered for any immobilized or bedridden individual with compromised skin integrity in order to prevent pressure sores from developing or to keep red, tender areas from deepening into serious wounds. Care is typically provided by specialized registered nurses called "enterostomal therapists" who are trained in skin and wound care as well as incontinence care and retraining, and care of individuals with surgically diverted urinary or fecal elimination (ostomy). A thorough risk assessment is conducted first and therapy is designed accordingly, employing specific wound care principles and practices shown to be effective for various levels of tissue injury.

Risk Assessment

Enterostomal therapists will note any conditions such as underlying disease, incontinence, or mental confusion that could impede pressure sore recovery. Nutritional status will be evaluated and a specific dietary plan may be designed to provide nutrition to benefit skin healing, including dietary supplements , intravenous (parenteral) feeding, restoring nitrogen balance and normal protein levels. Weight loss may be recommended for obese individuals. Pressure sores will be classified in one of four stages based on wound depth and skin condition: Stage I has intact skin with redness (erythema) and warmth; Stage II has loss of normal skin thickness, possible abrasion, swelling and blistering or peeling of skin; Stage III has full loss of normal skin thickness, an open wound (crater), and possible exposure of deeper layers of skin; Stage IV has full loss of normal skin thickness and erosion of underlying tissue extending into muscle, bone, tendon or joint, along with possible bone destruction, dislocation or pathologic fractures. Therapists will note if wounds are draining, if foul odors are present, or if any debris such as pieces of dead skin are in the wound. Presence of urine or feces from incontinence will be noted as well and regular care personnel will be advised about need for increased hygienic measures.

Pressure Relief

Reducing or eliminating pressure is the first task of wound care and requires the cooperation of the nursing center or family member responsible for onsite care. Recommendations will be made for shifting or turning the patient every two hours or other regular intervals. Some patients may benefit from lying flat on their backs; others may need the head of the bed lowered. Shear can be minimized by placing the patient on a special surface that alternates pressure points. A low-level of pressure relief can be obtained by using egg-crate mattresses or chair cushions. Egg-crate surfaces are constructed of sculpted foam with deep gullies between raised points of cushioning, which alternates pressure on vulnerable areas. Other types of air, foam and gel pressure-relieving surfaces are available. Wheel chair patients may need to be trained to shift their weight or lean side to side to relieve pressure. For deep wounds, burns, or pressure sore prevention, special "low air-loss" or "air-fluidized" beds are available that relieve pressure by constantly-moving air within specially designed pillows or within an entire bed surface filled with millions of tiny silicone-coated beads. Many institutions use beds that employ these principles to help heal wounds of all types and to prevent pressure sores from developing in at risk individuals.

Wounds First Aid

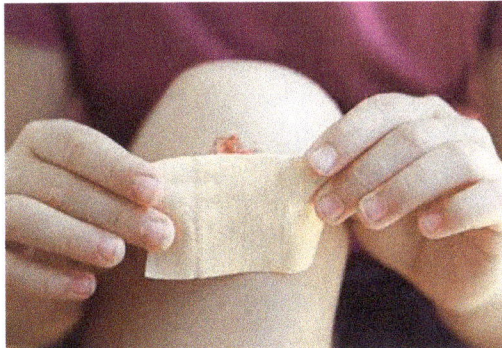

Wounds including minor cuts, lacerations, bites and abrasions can be treated with first aid. Given below are the steps to provide first aid to a wound:

1. Control bleeding

   Use a clean towel to apply light pressure to the area until bleeding stops (this may take a few minutes). Be aware that some medicines (e.g. aspirin and warfarin) will affect bleeding, and may need pressure to be applied for a longer period of time.

2. Wash your hands well

   Prior to cleaning or dressing the wound, ensure your hands are washed to prevent contamination and infection of the wound.

3. Rinse the wound

   Gently rinse the wound with clean, lukewarm water to cleanse and remove any fragments of dirt, e.g. gravel, as this will reduce the risk of infection.

4. Dry the wound

   Gently pat dry the surrounding skin with a clean pad or towel.

5. Replace any skin flaps if possible

   If there is a skin flap and it is still attached, gently reposition the skin flap back over the wound as much as possible using a moist cotton bud or pad.

6. Cover the wound

   Use a non-stick or gentle dressing and lightly bandage in place; try to avoid using tape on fragile skin to prevent further trauma on dressing removal.

7. Seek help

   Contact your general practitioner, nurse or pharmacist as soon as possible for further treatment and advice to ensure the wound heals quickly.

8. Manage pain

   Wounds can be painful, so consider pain relief while the wound heals. Talk to your GP about options for pain relief.

Wound Care Dressings

For more superficial Stage I and II pressure sores, treatment will involve keeping the wound clean and moist and the area around the sore clean and dry. Saline washes may be used and placement of sterile medicated non-stick gauze dressings that absorb wound drainage and fight infection-causing bacteria. Other bio-protective cleaning solutions include acetic acid, povidone iodine, and sodium hypochlorite. Harsh antiseptics, soaps and regular skin cleansers are not used because they can damage newly developing tissue. However, drying agents, lotions or ointments may be applied in a thin film over the wound three or four times daily. Massage of any at-risk area should be avoided because it encourages skin breakdown.

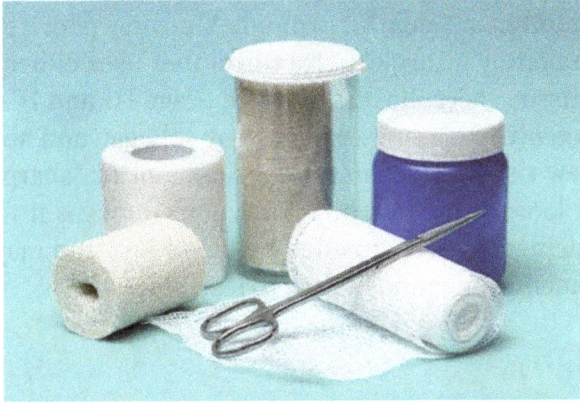

Whirlpool Treatment

Warm-water whirlpool treatments are sometimes used to treat pressure ulcers on arms, hands, feet or legs. This technique removes destroyed tissue fragments (necrotic tissue) by the force of irrigation followed by application of wet-to-dry non-stick dressings. After a wet dressing has been applied to the wound and allowed to dry, its removal picks up necrotic debris and a new dressing of sterile, medicated non-stick gauze or semi-permeable transparent adhesive dressings is applied to keep the area dry and prevent destruction of healthy skin near the wound, reducing risk of infection. Adhesive dressings are not recommended for draining wounds.

Hyperbaric Oxygen Therapy

Treatment of Stage III and IV decubitus ulcers, and other types of skin ulcers or burn wounds, may benefit from treatment that saturates the body with oxygen. The individual rests in a pressurized hyperbaric oxygen chamber, breathing 100% oxygen for 90 to 120 minutes. As the oxygen is absorbed by the blood, extra oxygen is provided to all cells and tissues, increasing healing capability and clearing of bacterial infection. Hyperbaric chambers are available in larger hospitals and medical centers.

Antimicrobial or Antibiotic Therapy

Antimicrobial topical therapy or oral antibiotic therapy may be recommended by the individual's physician to prevent possible bacterial infection or to address existing infection. Silver sulfadiazine is applied topically with good results. Antibiotics taken orally include penicillins, cephalospoins, aminoglycosides, sulfonamides, metronidazol and trimethoprim. Selection is based on specific bacteria causing infection or on obtaining the broadest possible coverage. Tissue biopsy may be performed to identify the causative bacteria.

Debridement and Debriding Agents

Surgical treatment is often needed for wounds showing poor response to standard wound care. Debridement is a surgical procedure that uses either a scalpel or chemicals to remove dead tissue (necrotic debris) from Stage III and IV wounds. Enzymatic debridement uses proteolytic enzymes that destroy collagen and necrotic wound debris without damaging new tissue. Mechanical debridement or "sharp debridement" perfomed with a scalpel loosens the necrotic tissue and removes it to encourage growth of new tissue. Debridement is accompanied by blood loss and may not be possible in individuals who are anemic or cannot afford to lose blood.

Urinary or Fecal Diversion

Incontinent individuals may require a surgical procedure (urinary or fecal diversion) to redirect the flow of urinary or fecal material to keep the wound clean, reducing likelihood of infection and encouraging positive response to medical treatment.

Reconstructive Surgery

Stage III and IV wounds may require consultation with a plastic surgeon to evaluate benefits of reconstructive surgery. Reconstructive surgery involves completely removing the ulcerated area and surrounding tissue (excision), debriding the bone, flushing the area with saline (lavage) to remove excess bacteria, and placing a drain in the wound for several days until risk of infection is gone and evidence of healing becomes apparent. Smaller wounds may then be sutured closed. Plastic surgery may follow surgical excision of a larger wound area, placing a flap of skin from another part of the body over the area to provide a new tissue surface. Skin grafts and other types of flaps may also be used for surgical closure (secondary closure) of excised wounds.

12

Patient Assistive Devices

Assistive technology can help to improve the quality of life for patients with diasbilities by allowing them greater independence for performing tasks that they cannot perform under normal circumstances. These technologies assist individuals with visual impairments, mobility impairments, eating impairments, etc. This chapter covers the use of patient assistive devices for walking, bathing, toileting, alternative communication devices, etc. and the role of nursing in assisting people who require such technologies.

Assistive devices are any piece of equipment that you can use to make your daily activities easier to perform. Some examples of assistive devices are wheelchairs, bath benches, as well as talking, hearing and vision aids.

Assistive devices can help you with,

- Walking
- Bathing
- Dressing
- Eating
- Speaking with family/friends, etc.

Many devices are commercially available (e.g. bath bench) or homemade by parents/family or health care professionals.

Some examples of assistive technologies are:

- People with physical disabilities that affect movement can use mobility aids, such as wheelchairs, scooters, walkers, canes, crutches, prosthetic devices, and orthotic devices, to enhance their mobility.

- Hearing aids can improve hearing ability in persons with hearing problems.

- Cognitive assistance, including computer or electrical assistive devices, can help people function following brain injury.

- Computer software and hardware, such as voice recognition programs, screen readers, and screen enlargement applications, help people with mobility and sensory impairments use computer technology.

- In the classroom and elsewhere, assistive devices, such as automatic page-turners, book holders, and adapted pencil grips, allow learners with disabilities to participate in educational activities.

- Closed captioning allows people with hearing impairments to enjoy movies and television programs.

- Barriers in community buildings, businesses, and workplaces can be removed or modified to improve accessibility. Such modifications include ramps, automatic door openers, grab bars, and wider doorways.

- Lightweight, high-performance wheelchairs have been designed for organized sports, such as basketball, tennis, and racing.

- Adaptive switches make it possible for a child with limited motor skills to play with toys and games.

- Many types of devices help people with disabilities perform such tasks as cooking, dressing, and grooming. Kitchen implements are available with large, cushioned grips to help people with weakness or arthritis in their hands. Medication dispensers with alarms can help people remember to take their medicine on time. People who use wheelchairs for mobility can use extendable reaching devices to reach items on shelves.

Assistive Devices for Walking

Mobility aids are often prescribed for individuals following a stroke to assist with safety, stability and muscle action when moving (e.g. walking). This equipment can assist the individual achieve greater independence. Mobility aids should be prescribed by a professional in order to meet the individual's own needs.

There are various mobility aids that are available including:

- Walking canes and walking sticks
- Roller walkers
- Wheelchairs
- Quad walkers.

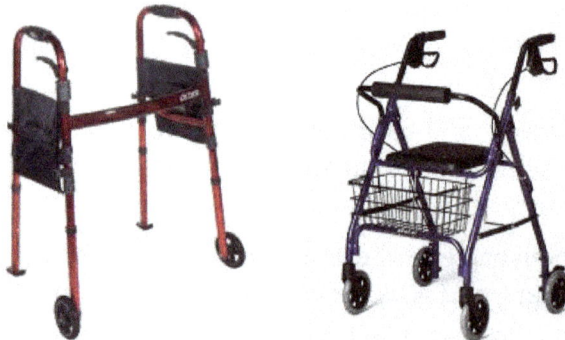

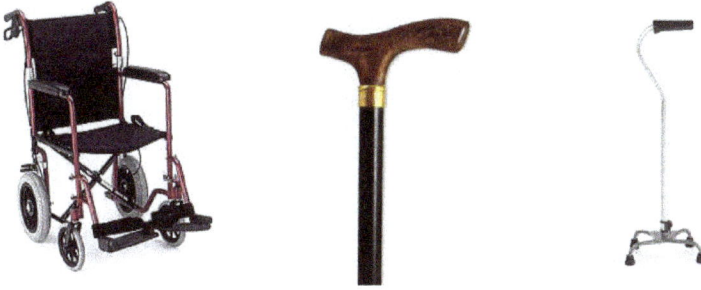

Assistive Devices for Bathing

Studies show that assistive devices often help people to be more independent. Everyone has their own bathing/showering habits and needs. Usually a combination of the following equipment is helpful.

Grab bars: Grab bars can be installed in the shower and/or next to the bathtub. Holding onto a grab bar will provide support when you:

- Stand up and sit down

- Go in and out of the shower or bathtub.

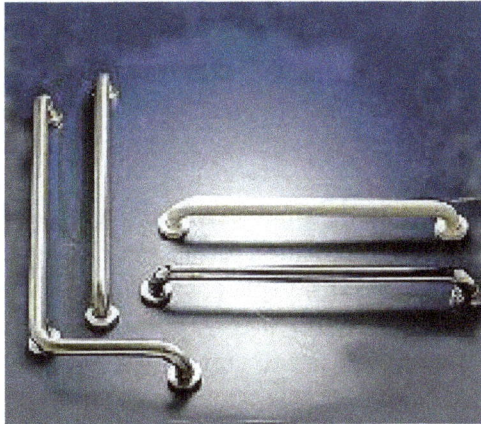

The number and type of grab bars depends on your needs. Some people only need one, others need more. This diagram shows some of the grab bars that are available. It is very important to install the grab bars firmly and at the right height or place to ensure your safety. You should talk to your occupational therapist or another health care professional for suggestions on the best way to install the bars. Grab bars can be installed onto the wall or clamped directly on the bathtub. Some bars may not be safe for you if you have a weak arm or leg caused by the stroke. Again, make sure to ask a health professional for help or advice before you purchase or install bars.

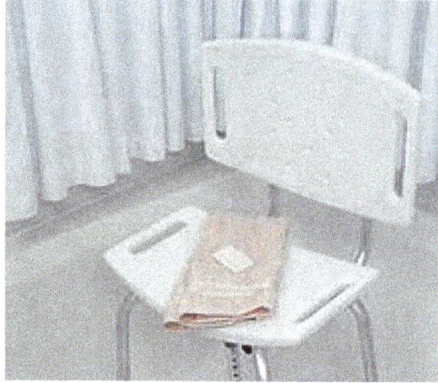

Bath chair/bench: A bath chair or bench allows you to sit during your bath or shower, which will save your personal energy levels. Sitting in the bath or shower is also a good idea if you are experiencing problems with balance.

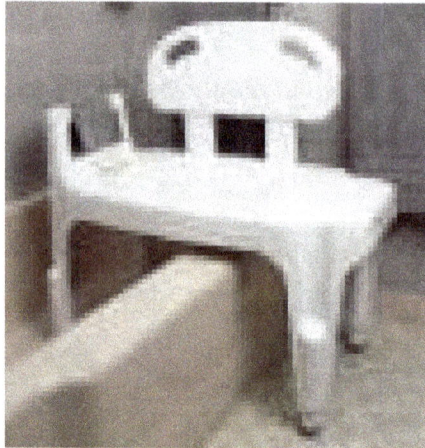

Transfer bath bench: A transfer bath bench can make it easier for you to get in and out of the bathtub. Once you are securely seated on the bench, you can lift your legs over the edge into the bathtub. Most people find this easier than lifting their leg over the edge of the bathtub while standing up. Again, it is important that a therapist or nurse show you the safest way to use this device before you try it on your own or with your family.

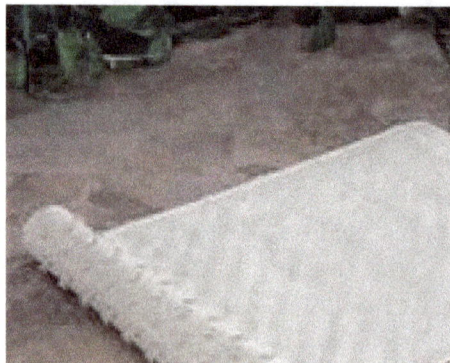

Anti-slip rubber mats: Anti-slip rubber mats placed inside and outside of the shower/ bathtub help prevent falls by providing a surface that is not slippery when it is wet.

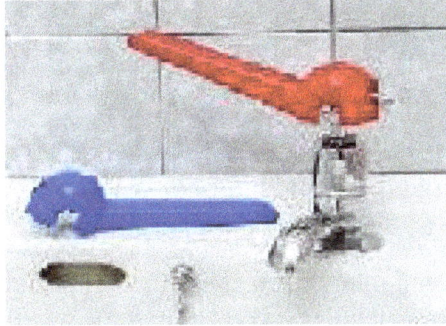

Tap turners: By adding leverage, tap turners make it easier for you to open and close taps. Long handle brushes and sponges: These devices provide assistance in washing parts of your body that require bending and stretching. Bath mitt: If you cannot use both hands it is often difficult to hold the soap, lather a washcloth, and wring it out.

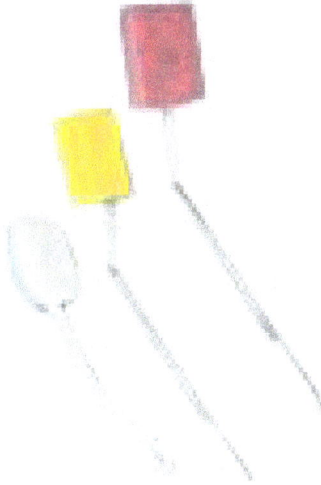

Assistive Devices for Toileting

Toileting is a task involving many steps:

- Entering the bathroom
- Getting on/off the toilet
- Managing clothing
- Cleaning yourself.

Each of these steps can represent a challenge for an individual who has had a stroke. The use of assistive devices can help you to perform these tasks more easily and more safely.

Bathroom Accessibility

Here are some guidelines to follow if you need to adapt your bathroom because it is not accessible for you:

- Ensure the doorframe is large enough for you to enter the bathroom easily, especially if you have a wheelchair or walker

- Ensure the space available within the bathroom allows you to circulate easily with a walker or a wheelchair (if you have one)

- Ensure the floor is free from unstable carpets that may cause you to slip and other objects to reduce the risks of falling.

If you cannot access the bathroom, there are other solutions available for you.

Urinals

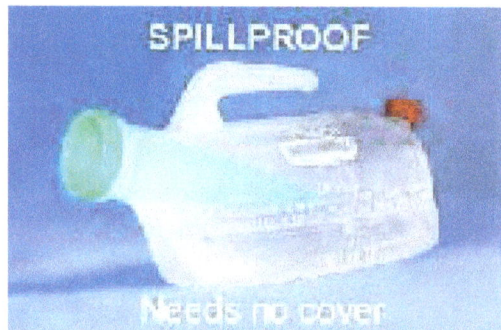

Urinals can be suitable for individuals who find it difficult to go in the bathroom or to transfer to the toilet. Urinals can be used in lying or sitting. They may be convenient for day and/or night use. Two types of urinals are available: male urinals (bottles) and female urinals. Urinals should not be use for bowel movement.

Bed Pans

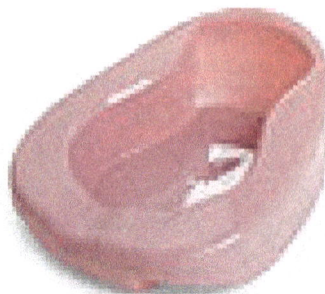

A bed pan can be used if you have difficulty getting up from your bed safely to go to the bathroom. Bed pans are designed to be used for bowel movements or urinating.

Bed pans and urinals should be washed regularly to prevent odors and for cleanliness.

Bedside Commode

A bedside commode can be used in the bedroom when it is difficult for you to access the bathroom or if you have difficulty reaching the bathroom on time. You can also use a urinal and/or a commode in another room.

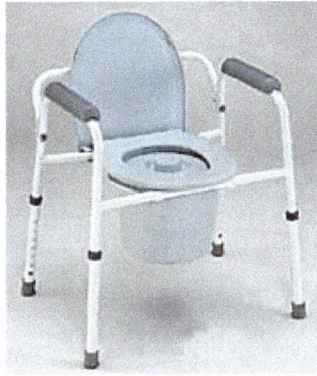

It is possible to adjust the height of a commode. It is important that your feet touch the ground (preferably flat) when you sit on the commode. Make sure that the breaks are on when transferring on to your commode. This will ensure safety and reduce the risks of injuries.

Getting On/Off the Toilet

There are also many assistive devices that make it easier to get on/off the toilet.

Fixed Grab Bars

Fixed grab bars are recommended for people who are able to walk into the bathroom and sit on the toilet while using only one hand for support. The grab bar has to be installed on a wall close to the toilet.

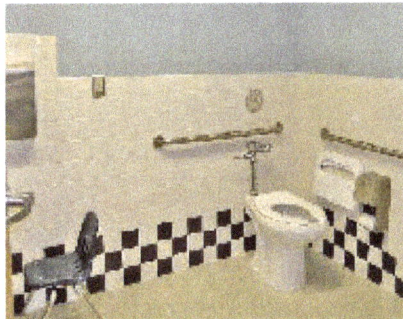

The most suitable types of grab bars and the ideal height of grab bars differ from one person to another. Consult an Occupational Therapist to ensure that the grab bar is installed correctly to suit your individual needs.

Fixed Toilet Frame

A toilet frame can be fixed to the floor around the toilet. This is suitable when there is no wall close to the toilet and/or the person needs two hands to hold on to something to get on/off the toilet.

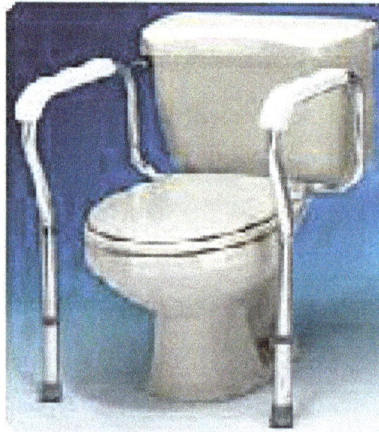

Raised Toilet Seat

A raised toilet seat increases the height of the toilet pan. This makes it easier to sit down on the toilet and stand up. Raised toilet seats of different heights are available commercially. The adequate height should allow the user to place his/her feet flat on the floor while seated on the toilet.

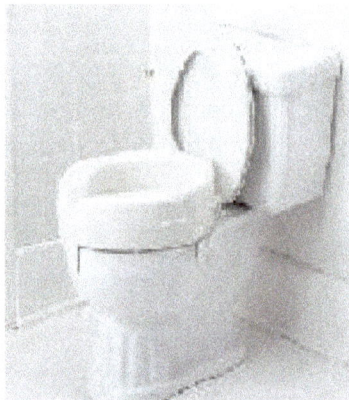

It is important to make sure that the raised toilet seat is securely attached to the toilet each time you use it. Incorrect fitting of the raised toilet seat increase risks of falls. It can also damage the seat if it is replaced incorrectly.

If you live with other people who use the same bathroom, they will need to know how to remove the raised toilet seat.

Toilet Frame with Seat / Toilet Seat with Handles

A toilet frame with seat or a toilet seat with handles provide both increased support and increased height. This can be useful for individuals who need a raised toilet seat and a toilet frame to help them move on and off the toilet.

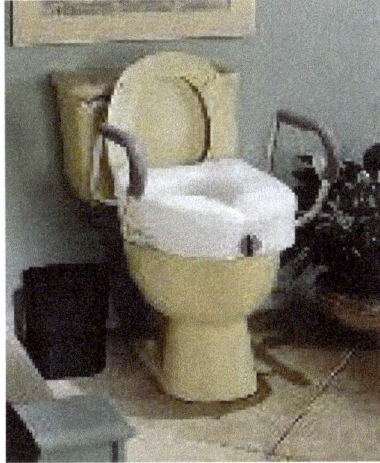

Cleaning yourself when using the Toilet

Sheets of Toilet Paper or Wet Wipe Sheets

If you have difficulty separating the sheets of a roll of toilet paper, consider using tissues, wet wipe sheets or toilet paper that has already been separated, as these options are easier to manipulate with one hand.

Portable Bidet/Bidet-toilets

If using toilet paper is very hard for you because you have difficulty moving one arm, you could use a bidet. However, these are not recommended if you have difficulty standing safely. Bidets are expensive devices.

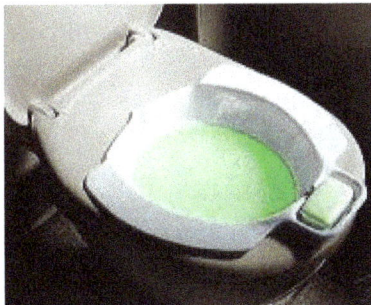

Assistive Devices for Eating

First, it is important for you to maintain a good position when eating. Sit in a chair that provides good support. If your trunk is weak and you need extra support, you can use pillows, an arm trough for your weaker arm, or a lap board. Good positioning will make it easier for you to swallow your food safely.

- Use cutlery: If it is difficult for you to use cutlery because one of your arms is weak, you can use adapted utensils which require the use of one hand.

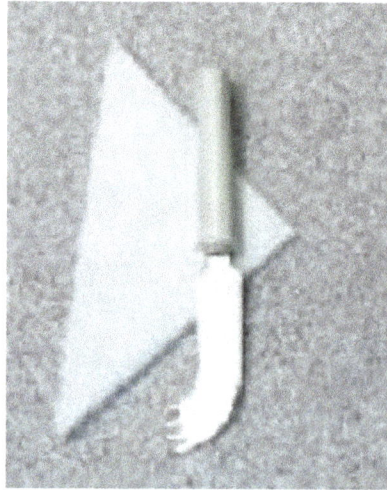

- Combined utensils (fork and knife, spoon and fork): Using these makes it so that you don't need to switch from one utensil to another. These utensils have been created for people who have one strong hand.

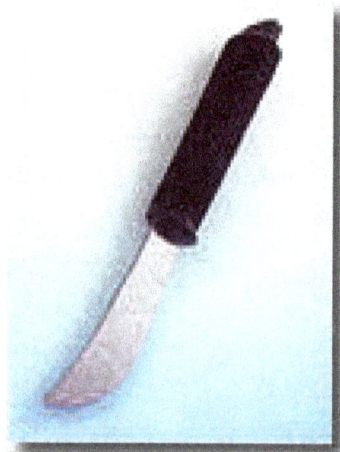

- Rocking knives: The rocking action prevents you from having to hold the food in place with the other hand allowing you to cut your food with only one hand.

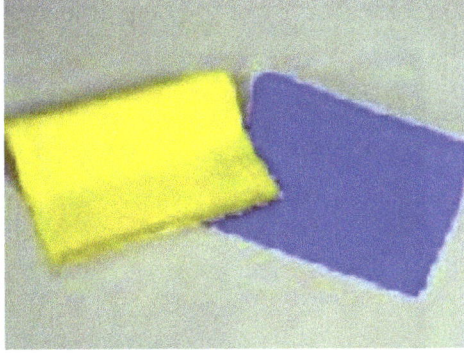

- Adhesive placemats: These hold the plate in place. People who have had a stroke often use only one hand when eating. Because they do not have the other hand to hold things down, the plate often moves during cutting or eating. By using a mat like the one in the picture, your plate will stay in one place.

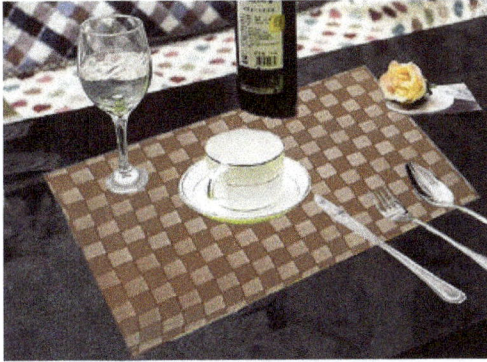

- Plate guards: These can help you use utensils without pushing food off of your plate. This is helpful for people who cannot use their second hand to hold the knife.

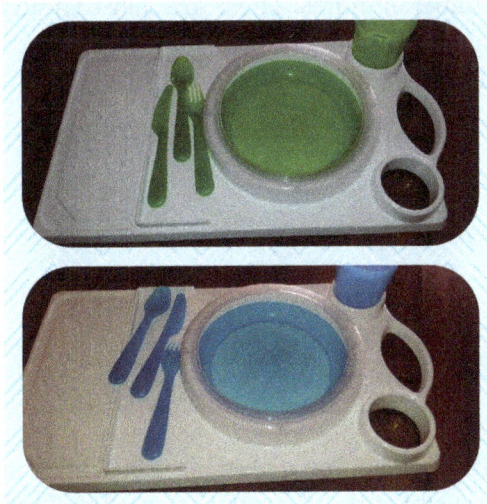

- Grasp objects: If it is difficult for you to grasp objects, you can try:

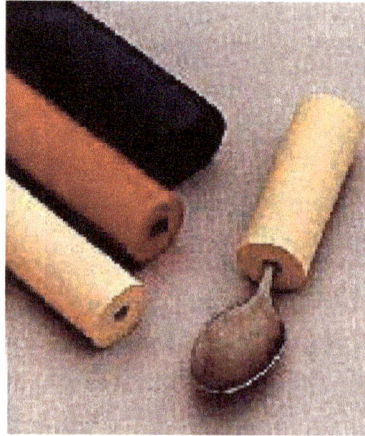

◦ Utensils with built-in or longer handles: If your hand is weak, these are easier to grasp.

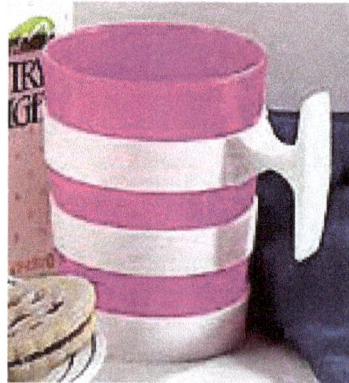

◦ Cups with T-shaped handles: These are easy to hold if you have trouble gripping, since you can simply put your fingers around the handle without closing your hand around it.

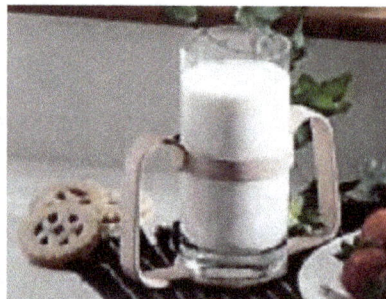

◦ Attachable handle to add on a glass or soft drink can: These can help you to hold a glass or a can without having to grasp it. They can be attached to any glass or can.

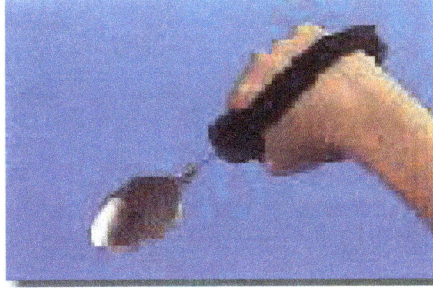

○   Universal cuff: These are to hold a utensil in place, making it easier for some individuals who have difficulty grasping utensils. It is possible to make the cuff tighter around your hand so that the utensil will not move.

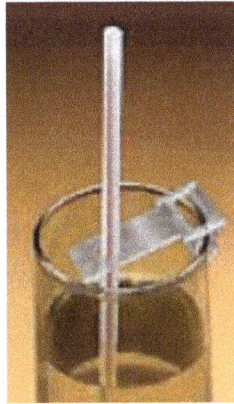

○   Drink from a glass or cup: The muscles that you use for drinking and swallowing may be weaker since your stroke. This can cause you to have difficulty drinking. If liquid is leaking out of your mouth when you drink, a straw might help you. You should talk to your health professional if you are having difficulty drinking. There are assessments that he or she will do to see if you are having problems with the muscles that are used for swallowing. A straw-holder may also make drinking easier for you as the straw is fixed into the glass and cannot fall out or move.

Alternative Communication Devices

When a child has a visual impairment and additional disabilities, she may need to use alternative methods to communicate her thoughts and needs. The child needs to have a variety of methods both to express her thoughts and to understand what others are communicating to her. The term "augmentative and alternative communication" (AAC) is used to refer to alternative communication methods that can support a child's efforts to communicate.

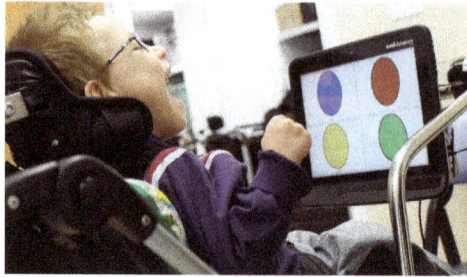

Augmentative and alternative communication methods can be unaided or aided, using objects or devices. Examples of unaided methods of communication include gestures, facial expressions, vocalizations, speech, and sign language(such as American Sign Language). Examples of aided forms of communication include the following:

- Using an actual object to convey meaning; for example, the child hands you a cup to let you know she is thirsty.

- Pointing to symbols, such as pictures or textures on a communication board or in a book.

- Activating a device; for example, the child presses a switch or button on a recorded speech device, initiating auditory output that says "I'm thirsty".

It is important for the child to have both aided and unaided methods of communication. Learning unaided methods of communication is important because a device or other communication aid may not always be available in every situation in which the child needs to communicate.

AAC Devices

Devices used for communication range from simple to sophisticated. There is a wide array of devices on the market, and they are continually changing. Every child's needs are different, and an AAC system is usually designed specifically for an individual child.

If the child is receiving special education services, her educational team will work with her to determine what devices may be most appropriate for her. It is important that one or more professionals who are familiar with communication issues be closely involved in this assessment. Such professionals might include a communication specialist—typically a speech therapist who has specialized in communication for children with significant communication issues—speech therapist, special educator, or occupational therapist.

It is equally important for the teacher of students with visual impairments to contribute to the selection of an AAC system by providing information about how the child uses any vision and other senses to obtain information from the world around her. The child will need different solutions depending on, for example, the size of the symbols she can see on a device, where in her visual field she needs to have the device positioned in order to see it, or whether she understands braille. If the child has useful vision, she should have a functional vision assessment to determine how she uses her vision before she is evaluated to see what kind of AAC system would best suit her needs.

The following are some broad categories of devices used by some children with visual impairments and additional disabilities.

- Communication board: A communication board can be made out of cardboard, wood, or another solid surface. Typically it has a grid on it with two or more symbols. The symbols can be concrete, such as actual objects or parts of objects; pictorial, such as photographs or drawings; alphabet symbols in print or braille; or words in print or braille. When using a communication board, a child can express herself by pointing to the symbol, picture, letters, or words that convey what she wants to share.

- Communication books: Like a communication board, a communication book has selected symbols that the child can point to in order to convey her message. The book may be arranged so that the first page has broad categories, such as emotions, foods, and people. Once the child picks a category, the person she is talking with turns to a page that offers more specific choices within that category.

- Recorded speech devices: With a recorded speech device, someone (such as you, a teacher, or a sibling) records messages for the child to use. The child activates the message using a switch or other button. Systems with multiple switches can store four, six, eight, or more messages. There are very complex AAC systems that enable the user to convey a wide array of information. For example, if the child has a device with four pre-recorded message slots, you might record four messages for bedtime, such as, "I want a blanket," "Read me another story," "I love you. Good night," and "Sit with me and rub my back." Once she is in bed, the child can press the appropriate switch or button to tell you what she wants.

- Keyboards: The child may type a message on a keyboard which then reads the message aloud. The symbols on the keyboard might be letters, words, or picture symbols.

References

- Assistive-devices-patient-info: strokengine.ca, Retrieved 09 July 2018

- Assistive-Devices-Patient-Family-brochure: strokengine.ca, Retrieved 17 March 2018

- Health, device, condition-info: nichd.nih.gov, Retrieved 15 July 2018

- Multiple-disabilities, communication, augmentative-and-alternative-communication-135: familyconnect.org, Retrieved 26 May 2018

Patient Nutrition

The nutrition of patients plays a crucial role in maintaining a healthy energy balance. It must be replete with the essential nutrients that speed up recovery. The routes of administration are oral, enteral or intravenous. This chapter studies the role of a nurse in patient nutrition and the basics of patient nutrition and hospital food.

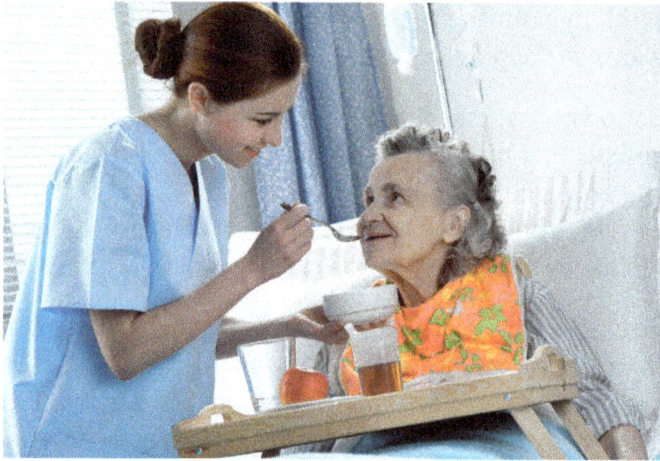

Nutrition has a significant impact on hospitalized patient outcomes and medical-surgical nurses are in a key position to lead in the delivery of effective nutrition care. The current era of health care delivery, with its focus on providing high-quality, affordable care, presents many challenges to hospital-based health professionals. The prevention and treatment of hospital malnutrition offers a tremendous opportunity to optimize the overall quality of patient care, improve clinical outcomes, and reduce costs. Unfortunately, malnutrition continues to go unrecognized and untreated in many hospitalized patients.

Clinical Nutrition

Clinical nutrition is the study of the relationship between food ingested and the well-being of the body.

More specifically, it is the science of nutrients and how they are digested, absorbed, transported, metabolised, stored, and utilised and how the resulting by-products are excreted as waste by the body. In addition to studying how food works in the body, nutritionists are interested in how the environment affects the quality and safety of foods, and how these factors influence heath and disease.

The actual study of human nutrition dates back to the 18th century, when the French chemist Antoine Lavoisier discovered that there was a relationship between metabolism of food and the process of breathing. Lavoisier, later crowned as "Father of Nutrition and Chemistry", demonstrated that oxidation of food is the source of body heat.

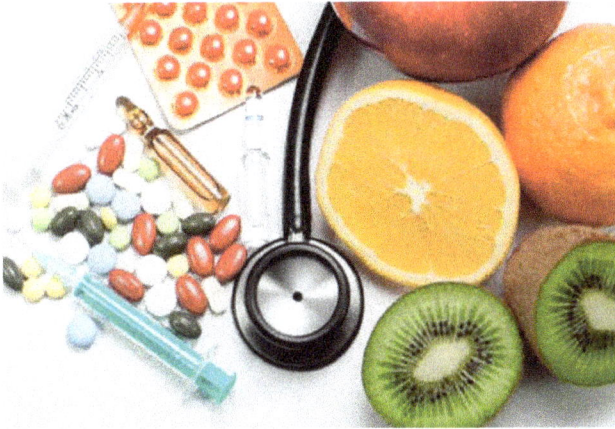

In the early 1940s Recommended Daily Allowances (RDAs) were established by the National Research Council, which established nutrition as a science on a national and international level. The RDAs defined the minimal nutrient intakes necessary for the prevention of Frank Deficiency States that are more likely to lead to severe deficiency diseases such as beri-beri and rickets. Until recently, these guidelines were used to set nutritional adequacy standards for the general population.

Researchers and scientists continue to uncover the therapeutic role of individual nutrients in the prevention and treatment of disease. For example antioxidants such as beta-carotene, selenium, vitamin E, and vitamin C appear to protect against the development of heart disease, cancer, and other chronic degenerative diseases.

The field of Clinical nutrition has evolved into a practice that is increasingly incorporated into mainstream medical treatment. Clinical nutrition is recognised as a modality that can enhance the well-being of a client during times of good health, ill health, and when undergoing conventional pharmaceutical protocols, as well as playing a vital role in disease prevention. "One size fits all" is no longer appropriate in determining the nutritional needs of an individual.

Clinical Nutritionist

A Clinical nutritionist has completed a minimum of 2 years training, including clinical assessment, holds an NZQA accredited, internationally recognized qualification and is registered with a local association that serves as an umbrella body.

A clinical nutritionist's recommendations will be based on the most recent research information combined with traditional experiential wisdom that has evolved over the centuries as to what foods should be eaten when and by whom.

Some may choose to see a clinical nutritionist as an adjunct to medical treatment to further enhance results or speed up recovery. Others may choose a nutritionist as their primary health care provider and the first port of-call for any health concern, trusting their practitioner will refer them on as needed. A clinical nutritionist may also help with prevention of ill health, helping establish a healthy lifestyle before any symptoms of imbalance manifest.

Hospital Food

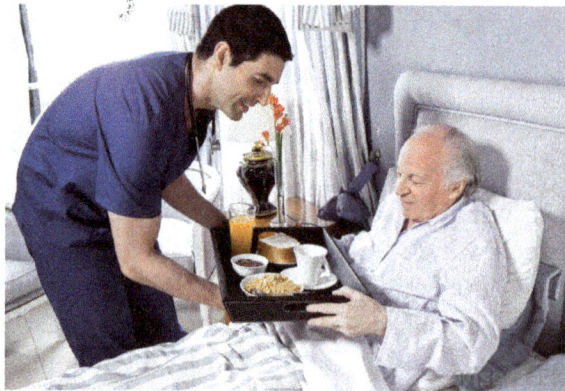

Food service in hospitals is often given a low priority instead of being recognised as an integral and important part of patient treatment and care. Up to now there have been no nationally agreed minimum guidelines for patients in acute hospitals.

Good nutrition is needed to ensure that the treatment the patient receives in hospital is as effective as possible. The number of patients who have good nutritional status, therefore, is a sound indicator of the quality of care provided by the hospital. It must be recognised that providing nutritious and appetising food is a key part of high-quality, effective hospital treatment.

Significant problems in the nutritional care and support of the undernourished and vulnerable patient include: limited food choice, the way food is served and lack of help for those unable to feed themselves properly. One major step in improving the food provided in hospitals is to ensure that hospital menus meet the needs of the patients; these menus should provide sufficient choice to offer adequate nutrition for all patients. The focus should be moved away from the production and serving of specific diets. Instead more attention should be given to frequent provision of appropriate energy-dense meals for undernourished patients.

Hospital Food Guidelines

- The standard menu for acute hospitals should be energy-dense and high-protein, providing at least 40% of energy from fat.

- A healthy-eating menu should be available for patients who are not malnourished or at risk of malnutrition. This menu should provide around 35% of energy from fat.

- A menu with at least 50% energy from fat should be available for patients with a poor appetite, high energy requirements and low food intake.

- Texture-modified menus should be available for patients with chewing or swallowing difficulties. These should provide at least 40% energy from fat.

- The standard menus must reach the minimum recommended daily amount (RDA) for protein and all vitamins and minerals.

- All menus must take into account the ethnic and religious needs of patients.

- All menus must, where possible, take into account patients' preferences.

- Patients must receive accurate descriptions of menu dishes to allow them to make informed choices. Picture menus must be available to aid patients with low literacy skills or poor vision.

- Menus must be developed in consultation with the hospital's clinical nutritionist/dietitian or the health board's clinical/community nutritionist/dietitian, the catering manager and the nutrition steering committee. Standard recipes should be used, where appropriate.

- Only evidence-based therapeutic diets should be prescribed.

- The nutritional status of the patient must be considered when therapeutic diets with a low fat content are indicated.

- The eating abilities and nutritional status of patients on texture-modified diets must be continually assessed.

- The clinical nutritionist/dietitian or physician should be aware of the patient's use of 'alternative diets' and the influence these might have on nutritional status.

- Feedback from patients about the acceptability of the food provided should be sought.

- The nutrient content and portion size of food should be audited per dish annually, or more often if the menu changes.

- In the planning stage, it should be documented that the nutrient content of the food is sufficient. This should be carried out in consultation with the clinical nutritionist/dietitian.

- Nutrient databases should be improved, with more reliable data on nutrient losses with different food-service systems.

Menu Composition

The guidelines below show the basic menus that every acute hospital should provide.

It is important to remember that normal low-fat, healthy-eating guidelines are not suitable for most patients in acute hospitals as such food will not provide enough concentrated energy to meet their needs.

Basic Menu Requirements

Below is a basic list of the minimum amounts of different foods each type of menu should provide to patients every day.

Where necessary, amounts of fruit and vegetables may be reduced on energy-dense menus, because fruit and vegetables are high in fibre and provide a feeling of satiety or fullness, thus reducing the appetite for other foods.

Since micronutrients may be lost during food preparation and requirements for some micronutrients may be higher in illness, it should be considered whether or not some patients might benefit from a vitamin-mineral supplement.

Table: Recommended minimum amounts of food which should be provided to each patient by the hospital menu

FOOD GROUP	DAILY INDIVIDUAL TARGETS	NOTES
Milk Fresh, whole milk	3 portions from this list daily: 1 portion is: 1/3 pint of milk 1oz of cheese Milk pudding or yoghurt	Whole milk should be used. Low-fat or skimmed milk should not be routinely used.
Meat, fish and alternatives Meat Poultry Fish Eggs Pulses	2 portions from this list daily: 1 portion is: 50-75g cooked weight 50-75g cooked weight 100-125g cooked weight 2 eggs per portion 75-100g beans served with 25g of cheese or 1 egg or 50g raw lentils	Halal meats should be available as appropriate; care must be taken not to contaminate non-halal meats with halal meats by using same utensils while cooking.

Starchy foods Breakfast cereals Bread Pasta Rice Potato	One or more of these foods at each meal. At least 6 portions daily. 1 portion is: 1 bowl of cereal 1 slice of bread 3 dessertspoons of pasta or rice 1 potato Number of portions daily depends on individual requirements.	
Fruit Fresh Dried Stewed Tinned Fruit juice	3 portions of fruit daily 1 portion is: 1 piece of fruit 1 fruit-based dessert e.g. apple tart/fruit salad 1 glass fruit juice	At least one portion of fruit should be in the form of fruit juice.
Vegetables Fresh Frozen	2 portions of vegetables daily. 1 portion is: 1 bowl of vegetable soup 2 tablespoons cooked vegetables 1 small salad	To prevent vitamin loss: • do not soak vegetables • do not add bicarbonate of soda • cook in minimal amount of water • cook in batches • cook until just tender and serve immediately after cooking Salad to include 3-4 vegetables Use a variety of vegetables.
Oils and spreads Butter Margarine Cooking oils	Butter and margarine should both be available. Foods can be fried in polyunsaturated or monounsaturated oils.	
Sugar Jam Marmalade Honey	Sugar, jam, honey and marmalade should be available to all nondiabetic patients.	
Fluids Tea Coffee Soup Fruit juice Water Squashes and soft drinks Milk	8 cups of fluid each day	

Menus

All menus should provide the minimum amounts as described above.

Standard Menu: high-protein, High-calorie

This high-protein, high-calorie menu is intended as the standard or normal menu in acute hospitals. Most patients in acute hospitals have higher energy needs than normal and may have smaller appetites. For this reason, the standard menu should provide 40% of energy from fat as this is a more concentrated source of calories.

Standard Menu Guidelines

- The standard menu is high-protein and high-calorie, providing 40% of energy from fat.

- This menu should provide two portion sizes: standard and large. The nutritional content of the menus should be as laid out in table below.

- Low-fat products should not be used (e.g. whole milk should be used instead of low-fat milk).

- Potatoes, vegetables and accompaniments to meals should be fortified with butter/oils (e.g. butter on potatoes and vegetables and oil dressings on salads).

- High-calorie desserts should be served and accompanied with a high-calorie sauce or dressing (e.g. ice cream, cream or custard). Desserts should be available at mid-day and evening meals.

- High-calorie snacks should be offered between meals.

Table: Macronutrient content of Standard Menu meal

	STANDARD PORTIONS	LARGE PORTIONS
Calories (kcal)	2000kcal	2500kcal
Protein (g)	90g	113g
Fat (g)	90g	110g

Table: Food amounts providing 7g of protein

FOOD	AMOUNT PROVIDING 7g PROTEIN
Lean meat (cooked)	28g
Fish	42g
Cheese	28g
Eggs	56g
Beans, peas, lentils	100g
Yoghurt	140g
Peanuts	28g
Milk	200ml

Table: Food amounts providing 2g of protein

FOOD	AMOUNT PROVIDING 2g PROTEIN
Bread	28g

Potato	112g
Breakfast cereal	28g
Flour	28g
Cooked rice	84g
Cooked pasta	70g

Healthy Eating Menu

A Healthy Eating menu should be available for patients with diabetes or high cholesterol and who are not malnourished or at risk of malnutrition. This menu should provide 35% energy from fat.

Energy-dense Menu

This menu should be available for patients with a very poor appetite and very low food intake.

Guidelines

- The aim of this menu is to provide small, frequent meals, which are high in energy and protein.

- The menu should provide 50% energy from fat. This can be achieved through high-calorie desserts and between-meal snacks or nourishing drinks.

- Low-fat products should not be used (e.g. whole milk should be used in place of low-fat milk).

- Potatoes, vegetables and accompaniments to meals should be fortified with butter/oils (e.g. butter on potatoes and vegetables and oil dressings on salads).

Suggestions for small, high-calorie meals for use with the energy dense menu.

- Milk pudding made with whole milk, with cream added

- Cream crackers with butter and cheddar cheese

- Chocolate mousse

- Fortified soup

- Sandwiches with meat fillings and mayonnaise

- Cheese on toast

- Trifle
- Chocolate

Texture-modified Menu

Texture-modified menus should be available for patients with chewing or swallowing difficulties. They should include set, pureed, semi-solid, soft or liquidised diets, as required by the patient. These menus should provide 40% energy from fat.

Guidelines

- Advice should be sought from a speech and language therapist about the appropriate consistency to use for each patient.
- If pureed meals are required, each part of the meal should be pureed separately.
- Food moulds should be used where possible for set/puree diets.
- Suitable food thickeners should be available for thickening fluids for set fluids.
- A nourishing liquid should be used when pureeing meals (e.g. milk, gravy, sauce, soup or custard).
- Meals may need to be fortified using high-protein/high-calorie powders.
- Between-meal nourishing snacks and nutritional drinks should be provided.

Special Menus

Special menus should be available for patients with conditions requiring a special menu – for example, coeliac or renal disease. The particular menus used should be selected by the hospital in accordance with the patient's requirements. All menus should meet the basic nutritional requirements described above.

Meal Pattern

Hospital mealtimes are often inflexible and designed to meet the needs of staff rather than those of patients:

- Meals are often close together, with long fasts between the evening meal and breakfast.
- Ward rounds and diagnostic procedures often interrupt mealtimes.

In-between meals and snacks increase total food consumption.

Guidelines

- Three main meals should be served daily: breakfast, lunch and dinner.

- Nourishing snacks and drinks should be served between meals: mid-morning, mid-afternoon and late-evening. They should also be available on the wards at all times and be routinely offered to patients who miss meals and snacks.

- There should be four hours or more between the end of each main meal and the beginning of the next.

- The mealtimes should be spread to cover most of the waking hours.

- Patients should be given adequate time to eat their meals.

- Interruption of patients' mealtimes by ward rounds and diagnostic procedures should be minimised. Hospitals are encouraged to have 'protected mealtimes' to allow patients to eat undisturbed.

- Snacks and nourishing drinks between meals should be offered routinely.

- A range of nourishing food supplements, such as fortified drinks and soups, should be available on every ward.

- The use of sip feeding should be targeted and supervised properly. Sip feeds should be prescribed by the clinical nutritionist/dietician and dispensed by the nurses on the medication rounds. A nutrition supplement-monitoring chart should be designed and used.

Serving Meals

Guidelines

- Meals should be served at the correct temperature – hot foods should be hot and cold foods should be cold.

- Where patients are eating in bed, trays should be placed close enough for the patient to reach comfortably, especially in the case of incapacitated patients.

- Tray and dish covers should be removed for incapacitated patients.

- Where required, modified cutlery and other feeding aids must be given to the patient before serving the meal.

- Where assistance with feeding is required, the assistant must be available at the time the meal is served.

- Responsibility for feeding patients should be clearly assigned.

Monitoring Food Intake

Guidelines

- The nursing staff is responsible for overseeing the monitoring of the food intake of patients on their wards.

- Tray collection should be supervised closely to enable monitoring of patients' food intake.

- The food intake of all patients should be registered by means of a semi-quantitative system.

- The food intake of all patients at nutritional risk and receiving nutritional support should be registered by means of dietary records.

- Information from the catering department about the portion size and energy content of hospital food should be available, to aid ward personnel in noting the food intake of patients.

- The appropriate personnel on the wards should be trained in how to monitor food intake.

- The information about patients' food intake should be used to develop appropriate menus for specific groups.

- A system to monitor food wastage should be implemented.

- Studies should be undertaken to develop and validate simple food-registration methods.

Role of a Nurse in Patient Nutrition

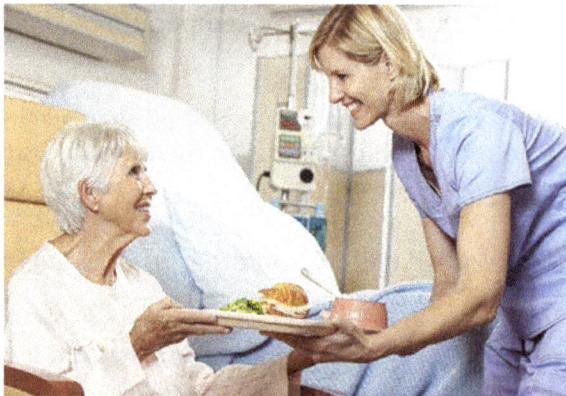

There are many ways nurses can teach their patients about proper nutrition as it relates to their health. Presentations at community health centers are crucial to community health. A nurse with the right knowledge can prepare a PowerPoint presentation to show for a group of seniors during a health fair. They can also give the attendees literature to take home for further study and guidance. Similarly, a school nurse can present students with the facts about healthy nutrition during a school assembly as well as giving them brochures to take home.

Nurses who work in hospitals and clinics are likely more concerned with nutrition as it relates to recovery from illness, surgery or other treatments. Nurses can talk to patients at the bedside and explain the special meals they have at the hospital that aid recovery, as many patients will be on special diets during their stay. These nurses can also gather informative and accurate literature to give patients when they are discharged. Healthy eating goes far beyond the hospital, especially if the patient plans to stay out of the hospital.

Perioperative Care

Perioperative care is the care provided to a patient before, during and after a patient's surgical procedure. Accordingly, it is divided into preoperative, peroperative and post-operative care. This chapter explores the essentials of perioperaive care and the role of nurses during the perioperative period.

Perioperative Period

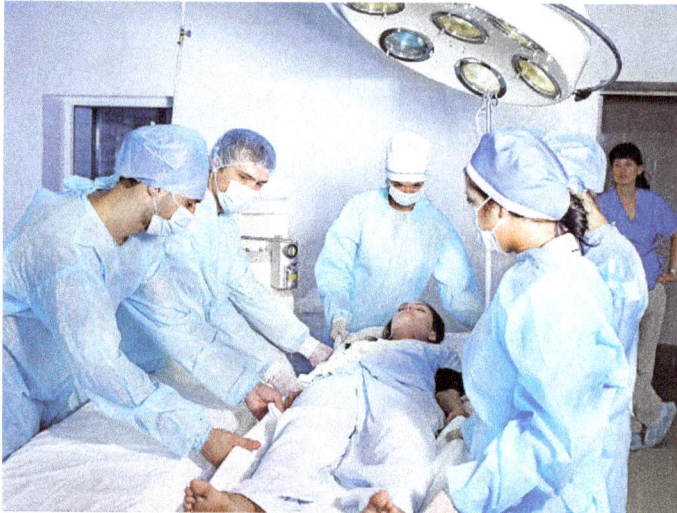

The perioperative period is a term used to describe the three distinct phases of any surgical procedure, which includes the preoperative phase, the intraoperative phase, and the postoperative phase.

Every surgery is broken down into these phases to differentiate tasks and establish who is responsible for overseeing and delivering each stage of care. By maintaining a strict adherence to procedures and a clear chain of command, hospital teams are able to deliver consistent, optimal care from the moment a surgery is ordered to the time when a person is fully recovered.

Preoperative Phase

The initial phase, called the preoperative phase, begins with the decision to have surgery and ends when the patient is wheeled into surgery. This phase can be extremely brief, such as in the cases of acute trauma, or require a long period of preparation during which time a person may be required to fast, lose weight, undergo preoperative tests, or await the receipt of an organ for transplant.

One of the goals of the preoperative phase is to manage the anxiety that may arise, either as result of an emergency situation or having to wait for inordinately long periods of time. Preoperative anxiety is a common reaction experienced by patients and one that can be relieved with on-going interaction with one or more members of the medical team.

Prior to intake, that person will usually be the treating doctor and/or surgeon. Once a person is admitted into a hospital, patient care and oversight will typically be coordinated by one or several perioperative nurses.

Intraoperative Phase

The second phase, known as the intraoperative phase, involves the surgery itself. It starts when the patient is wheeled into the surgical suite and ends when the patient is wheeled to the post-anesthesia care unit (PACU).

During this phase, the patient will be prepped and typically given some form of anesthesia, either general anesthesia (for complete unconsciousness), local anesthesia (to prevent pain while awake), or regional anesthesia (such as with a spinal or epidural block).

As the surgery begins, the patient's vital signs (including heart rate, respiration, and blood oxygen) will be closely monitored. In addition to the roles of the surgeon and anesthesiologist, other team members will be responsible for assisting the surgeon, ensuring safety, and preventing infection during the course of the surgery.

Postoperative Phase

The final phase, known as the postoperative phase, is the period immediately following surgery. As with the preoperative phase, the period can be brief, lasting a few hours, or require months of rehabilitation and recuperation.

Once the patient is awake and ready to leave PACU, the post-anesthesia nurse will typically transfer the responsibility of care back to the perioperative nurse. (In smaller hospitals, the same person may be tasked with both responsibilities.)

Postoperative care is mainly focused on monitoring and managing the patient's physiological health and aiding in the post-surgical recovery. This may include ensuring hydration, monitoring urination or bowel movements, assisting with mobility, providing appropriate nutrition, managing pain, and preventing infection.

Perioperative Nurse

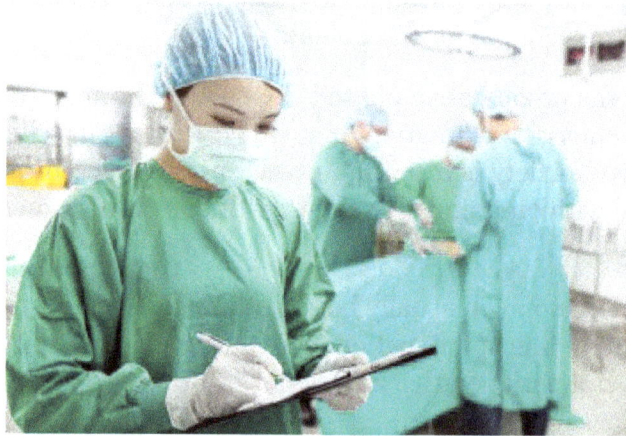

Perioperative nurses help plan, carry out, and assess treatment for patients undergoing surgery. Working in hospital surgical departments, ambulatory surgery units, clinics, or physicians' offices, these RNs are involved in the care of patients before, during, and after surgery.

Types of perioperative nurses include the following:

- A scrub nurse is sterile and is responsible for choosing and handling instruments and supplies used during surgery. Duties include setting up a sterile area in preperation for surgery, helping the surgical team with gowns and gloves, and handing instruments to the surgeon.

- The duties of a circulating nurse include developing a patient plan of care, reviewing preoperative assessments with patients, and managing activities in the operating room. The circulating nurse is not sterile, but is there to serve everyone involved in a surgical procidure, not just the surgeon.

- The RN first assistant (RNFA) assists during the operation by helping with surgical activities such as keeping bleeding under control, exposing wounds, and suturing, all under direction of the surgeon. Becoming an RNFA requires additional training beyond basic perioperative training.

- A PACU (Post Anesthesia Care Unit) RN cares for patients immediately after surgical procedures and anesthesia.

15

Reproduction Care

The care of pregnant mothers prior to childbirth, during and after childbirth is essential to her health and safety as well as that of the newborn. Neonatal nursing or care for infants is a specialty of nursing care. Dealing with prematurity, infection, birth defects, surgical and cardiac malformations are also part of neonatal care. Nurses are vital to the deliverance of reproduction care and neonatal care. This chapter has been written to provide an extensive understanding of reproduction care and neonatal care and the role of nursing in providing it.

Reproductive Health

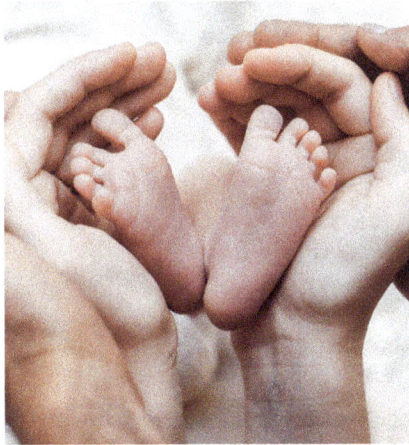

Reproductive health is a state of complete physical, mental and social well-being and not merely the absence of disease or infirmity, in all matters relating to the reproductive system and to its functions and processes. Reproductive health therefore implies that people are able to have a satisfying and safe sex life and that they have the capability to reproduce and the freedom to decide if, when and how often to do so.

Implicit in this last condition are the rights of men and women to be informed and to have access to safe, effective, affordable and acceptable methods of family planning of their choice, as well as other methods of their choice for regulation of fertility which are not against the law, and the right of access to appropriate health care services that will enable women to go safely through pregnancy and childbirth and provide couples with the best chance of having a healthy infant.

In line with the above definition of reproductive health, reproductive health care is defined as the constellation of methods, techniques and services that contribute to reproductive health and well-being by preventing and solving reproductive health problems. It includes maternal and perinatal health, family planning, preventing unsafe abortion, prevention and treatment of sexually transmitted diseases and promoting sexual health.

Adolescent Health

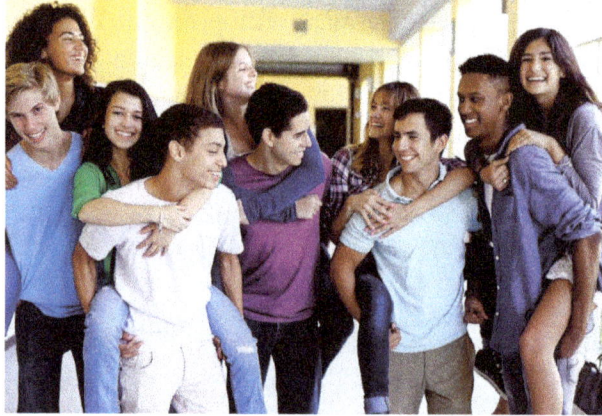

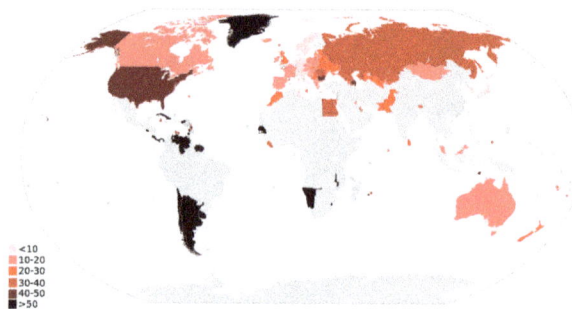

Teenage birth rate per 1,000 females aged 15–19

Adolescent health creates a major global burden and has a great deal of additional and diverse complications compared to adult reproductive health such as early pregnancy and parenting issues, difficulties accessing contraception and safe abortions, lack of healthcare access, and high rates of HIV and sexually transmitted infections, and mental health issues. Each of those can be affected by outside political, economic and socio-cultural influences. For most adolescent females, they have yet to complete their body growth trajectories, therefore adding a pregnancy exposes them to a predisposition to complications. These complications range from anemia, malaria, HIV and other STI's, postpartum bleeding and other postpartum complications, mental health disorders such as depression and suicidal thoughts or attempts. In 2014, adolescent birth rates between the ages of 15-19 was 44 per 1000, 1 in 3 experienced sexual violence, and there more than 1.2 million deaths. The top three leading causes of death in females between the ages of 15-19 are maternal conditions 10.1%, self-harm 9.6%, and road conditions 6.1%.

The causes for teenage pregnancy are vast and diverse. In developing countries, young women are pressured to marry for different reasons. One reason is to bear children to help with work, another on a dowry system to increase the families income, another is due to prearranged marriages. These reasons tie back to financial needs of girls' family, cultural norms, religious beliefs and external conflicts.

Adolescent pregnancy, especially in developing countries, carries increased health risks, and contributes to maintaining the cycle of poverty. The availability and type of sex education for teenagers varies in different parts of the world. LGBT teens may suffer additional problems if they live in places where homosexual activity is socially disapproved and/or illegal; in extreme cases there can be depression, social isolation and even suicide among LGBT youth.

Maternal Health

Ninety nine percent of maternal deaths occur in developing countries and in 25 years, maternal mortality globally dropped to 44%. Statistically, a woman's chance of survival during childbirth is closely tied to her social economic status, access to healthcare, where she lives geographically, and cultural norms. To compare, a woman dies of complications from childbirth every minute in developing countries versus a total of 1% of total maternal mortality deaths in developed countries. Women in developing countries have little access to family planning services, different cultural practices, have lack of information, birthing attendants, prenatal care, birth control, postnatal care, lack of access to health care and are typically in poverty. In 2015, those in low-income countries had access to antenatal care visits averaged to 40% and were preventable. All these reasons lead to an increase in the Maternal Mortality Ratio (MMR).

One of the international sustainable development goals developed by United Nations is to improve maternal health by a targeted 70 deaths per 100,000 live births by 2030. Most models of maternal health encompass family planning, preconception, prenatal, and postnatal care. All care after childbirth recovery is typically excluded, which includes pre-menopause and aging into old age. During childbirth, women typically die from severe bleeding, infections, high blood pressure during pregnancy, delivery complications, or an unsafe abortion. Other reasons can be regional such as complications related to diseases such as malaria and AIDS during pregnancy. The younger the women is when she gives birth, the more at risk her and her baby is for complications and possibly mortality.

Contraception

Access to reproductive health services is very poor in many countries. Women are often unable to access maternal health services due to lack of knowledge about the existence of such services or lack of freedom of movement. Some women are subjected to forced pregnancy and banned from leaving the home. In many countries, women are not allowed to leave home without a male relative or husband, and therefore their ability to access medical services is limited. Therefore, increasing women's autonomy is needed in order to improve reproductive health, however doing may require a cultural shift. According to the WHO, "All women need access to antenatal care in pregnancy, skilled care during childbirth, and care and support in the weeks after childbirth".

The fact that the law allows certain reproductive health services, it does not necessary ensure that such services are *de facto* available to people. The availability of contraception, sterilization and abortion is dependent on laws, as well as social, cultural and religious norms. Some countries have liberal laws regarding these issues, but in practice it is very difficult to access such services due to doctors, pharmacists and other social and medical workers being conscientious objectors.

About 220 million women worldwide have an unmet need for birth control. The updated contraceptive guidelines in South Africa are attempting to improve access by providing special service delivery and access considerations for the following: sex workers, lesbian, gay, bisexual, transgender and intersex individuals, migrants, men, adolescents, women who are perimenopausal, those who have a disability or chronic condition. They also aim to increase access to long acting contraceptive methods, particularly the copper IUD, the introductions of single rod progestogen implant, and combined estrogen and progestogen injectables. The copper IUD has been provided significantly less frequently than other contraceptive methods but signs of an increase in most provinces were reported. The most frequently provided method was injectable progesterone, due to ease of administration, which acknowledged was not ideal as the injection last only months, and emphasised condom use with this method because it can increase the risk of HIV: The product made up 49% of South Africa's contraceptive use and up to 90% in some provinces.

Tanzanian provider perspectives address the obstacles to consistent contraceptive use in their communities. It was found that the capability of dispensaries to service patients was determined by inconsistent reproductive goals, low educational attainment, misconceptions about the side effects of contraceptives, and social factors such as gender dynamics, spousal dynamics, economic conditions, religious norms, cultural norms, and constraints in supply chains. A provider referenced and example of propaganda spread about the side effects of contraception: "There are influential people, for example elders and religious leaders. They normally convince people that condoms contain some microorganisms and contraceptive pills cause cancer". Another said that women often had pressure from their spouse or family that caused them to use birth control secretly or to discontinue use, and that women frequently preferred undetectable methods for this reason. Access was also hindered as a result of a lack in properly trained medical personnel: "Shortage of the medical attendant...is a challenge, we are not able to attend to a big number of clients, also we do not have enough education which makes us unable to provide women with the methods they want". The majority of medical centers were staffed by people without medical training with few doctors and nurses, despite federal regulations, due to lack of resources. One center had only one person who was able to insert and remove implants, and without her they were unable to service people who wanted an implant inserted or removed.

Another dispensary that carried two methods of birth control shared that they sometimes run out of both materials at the same time. Constraints in supply chains sometimes cause dispensaries to run out of contraceptive materials. Providers also claimed that more male involvement and education would be helpful and perhaps allow more females to stay compliant on birth control.

Sexually Transmitted Infection

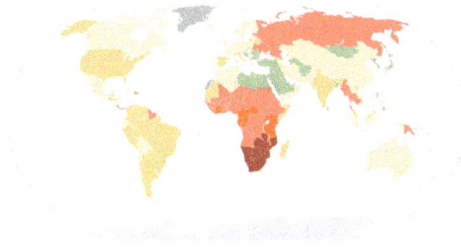

Estimated prevalence in % of HIV among young adults (15–49) per country

A Sexually transmitted infection (STI) previously known as a *sexually transmitted disease (STD)* or *venereal disease (VD)* is an infection that has a significant likelihood of transmission between humans by means of sexual activity. The CDC analyses the eight most common STI's: chlamydia, gonorrhea, hepatitis B virus (HBV), herpes simplex virus type 2 (HSV-2), human immunodeficiency virus (HIV), human papillomavirus (HPV), syphilis, and trichomoniasis.

There are more than 600 million cases of STI's worldwide and more than 20 million new cases within the United States. Numbers of such high magnitude weigh a heavy burden on the local and global economy. A study conducted at Oxford University in 2015 concluded that despite giving participants early antiviral medications (ART), they still cost an estimated $256 billion over 2 decades. HIV testing done at modest rates could reduce HIV infections by 21%, HIV retention by 54% and HIV mortality rates by 64%, with a cost-effectiveness ration of $45,300 per Quality-adjusted life year. However, the study concluded that the United States has led to an excess in infections, treatment costs, and deaths, even when interventions do not improve over all survival rates.

There is a profound reduction on STI rates once those who are sexually active are educated about transmissions, condom promotion, interventions targeted at key and vulnerable populations through a comprehensive Sex education courses or programs. South Africa's policy addresses the needs of women at risk for HIV and who are HIV positive as well as their partners and children. The policy also promotes screening activities related to sexual health such as HIV counseling and testing as well as testing for other STIs, tuberculosis, cervical cancer, and breast cancer.

Young African American women are at a higher risk for STI's, including HIV. A recent study published outside of Atlanta, Georgia collected data (demographic, psychological, and behavioral measures) with a vaginal swab to confirm the presence of STIs. They found a profound difference that those women who had graduated from college were far less likely to have STIs, potentially be benefiting from a reduction in vulnerability to acquiring STIs/HIV as they gain in education status and potentially move up in demographic areas and/or status.

Abortions

In articles from the World Health Organization, it claims that legal abortion is a fundamental right of women regardless of where they live and unsafe abortion is a silent pandemic. In 2005, it was estimated that 19-20 million abortions had complications, some complications are permanent, while another estimated 68,000 women died from unsafe abortions. Having access to safe abortion can have positive impacts on women's health and life, and vice versa. Legislation of abortion on request is necessary but an insufficient step towards improving women's health. In some countries where it abortion is legal, and has been for decades, there has been no improvement in access to adequate services making abortion unsafe due to lack of healthcare services. It is hard to get an abortion due to legal and policy barriers, social and cultural barriers (gender discrimination, poverty, religious restrictions, lack of support etc., health system barriers (lack of facilities or trained personnel), however safe abortions with trained personnel, good social support, and access to facilities, can improve maternal health and increase reproductive health later in life.

The WHO's Development and Research Training in Human Reproduction (HRP), whose research concerns people's sexual and reproductive health and lives, has an overall strategy to combat unsafe abortion that comprises four inter-related activities:

- To collate, synthesize and generate scientifically sound evidence on unsafe abortion prevalence and practices;

- To develop improved technologies and implement interventions to make abortion safer;

- To translate evidence into norms, tools and guidelines;

- To assist in the development of programmes and policies that reduce unsafe abortion and improve access to safe abortion and high quality post-abortion care.

During and after the International Conference on Population and Development (ICPD), some interested parties attempted to interpret the term 'reproductive health' in the sense that it implies abortion as a means of family planning or, indeed, a right to abortion. These interpretations, however, do not reflect the consensus reached at the Conference. For the European Union, where legislation on abortion is certainly less restrictive than elsewhere, the Council Presidency has clearly stated that the Council's commitment to promote 'reproductive health' did not include the promotion of abortion. Likewise, the European Commission, in response to a question from a member of the European Parliament, clarified:The term 'reproductive health' was defined by the United Nations (UN) in 1994 at the Cairo International Conference on Population and Development. All Member States of the Union endorsed the Programme of Action adopted at Cairo. The Union has never adopted an alternative definition of 'reproductive health' to that given in the Programme of Action, which makes no reference to abortion.

The term 'reproductive health' was defined by the United Nations (UN) in 1994 at the Cairo International Conference on Population and Development. All Member States of the Union endorsed the Programme of Action adopted at Cairo. The Union has never adopted an alternative definition of 'reproductive health' to that given in the Programme of Action, which makes no reference to abortion.

A few days prior to the Cairo Conference, Vice President Al Gore, stated for the record:

> "Let us get a false issue off the table: the US does not seek to establish a new international right to abortion, and we do not believe that abortion should be encouraged as a method of family planning".

Some years later, the position of the US Administration in this debate was reconfirmed by US Ambassador to the UN, Ellen Sauerbrey, when she stated at a meeting of the UN Commission on the Status of Women that:

> "Nongovernmental organizations are attempting to assert that Beijing in some way creates or contributes to the creation of an internationally recognized fundamental right to abortion. There is no fundamental right to abortion. And yet it keeps coming up largely driven by NGOs trying to hijack the term and trying to make it into a definition".

Contraception prevents 112 million abortions per year by UN estimates Abortion is declining in all age groups but still a global pandemic.

Female Genital Mutilation/Circumcision

Female genital mutilation (FGM) or female genital circumcision or cutting is most commonly known as the complete or partial removal of the external female genitalia or other injury to female genital organs for a non-medical reason. This is mostly practiced in around 30 countries and affecting around 160 million women and girls, globally, and between 500,000 and 515,000 in the United States.

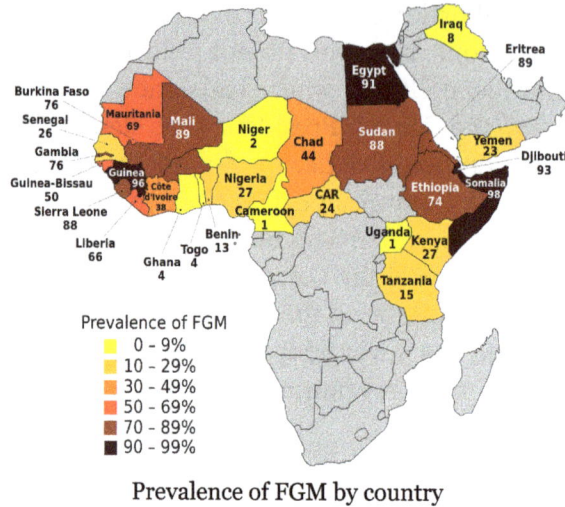

Prevalence of FGM by country

There are four types:

- Cliteridectomy: partial or total removal of the clitoris (a small, sensitive and erectile part of the female genitals) and/or in very rare cases only, the prepuce (the fold of skin surrounding the clitoris).

- Excision: partial or total removal of the clitoris and the labia minora, with or without excision of the labia majora (the labia are the 'lips' that surround the vagina).

- Infibulation: narrowing of the vaginal opening through the creation of a covering seal. The seal is formed by cutting and re-positioning the inner, or outer, labia, with or without removal of the clitoris.

- Other: all other harmful procedures to the female genitalia for non-medical purposes (piercing, scraping, cauterizing of the genital area).

There are no health benefits of FGM, as it interferes with the natural functions of a woman's and girls' bodies, such as causing severe pain, shock, hemorrhage, tetanus or sepsis (bacterial infection), urine retention, open sores in the genital region and injury to nearby genital tissue, recurrent bladder and urinary tract infections, cysts, increased risk of infertility, childbirth complications and newborn deaths. Sexual problems are 1.5 more likely to occur in women who have undergone FGM, they may experience painful intercourse, have less sexual satisfaction, and be two times more likely to report lack of sexual desire. In addition, the maternal and fetal death rate is significantly higher due to childbirth complications.

The psychological effects of FGM can cause severe trauma throughout women's lives. 80% of the studies showed that women have PTSD or other such psycho-affective disorders. Other women identified with socio-cultural differences in the meaning of "consequences".

An additional study, including 66 immigrant women in the Netherlands regarding the impact genital cutting can have on mental health was conducted. The women were given four tests: the Harvard Trauma Questionnaire-30, Hopkins Symptom Checklist-25, COPE-easy, and Lowlands Acculturation Scale. The participants were between the ages of 18 and 69, with an average age of 35.5, 43% of participants were married, and 79% of participants had children. Thirty-six of the participants had experienced a type 3 mutilation, 9 experienced a type 2 mutilation, and 21 experienced a type one mutilation. The study found that 33.3% of the women were above the cut off for an affective or anxiety disorder and PTSD was indicated by 17.5% of participant score. The study also found that PTSD was more likely in those who experienced the type 3 mutilation had vivid memories of the event, and who used abused substances to cope. It was also found that with type 3 mutilations, substance misuse, avoidance coping, and lack of money were associated with those who experienced depression and anxiety.

HIV/AIDS in Africa is a major public health problem. Sub-Saharan Africa is the worst affected world region for prevalence of HIV, especially among young women. 90% of the children in the world living with HIV are in sub-Saharan Africa.

In most African countries, the total fertility rate is very high, often due to lack of access to contraception and family planning, and practices such as forced and child marriage. Niger, Angola, Mali, Burundi and Somalia have very high fertility rates.

The updated contraceptive guidelines in South Africa attempt to improve access by providing special service delivery and access considerations for sex workers, lesbian, gay, bisexual, transgender and intersex individuals, migrants, men, adolescents, women who are perimenopausal, have a disability, or chronic condition. They also aim to increase access to long acting contraceptive methods, particularly the copper IUD, and the introductions of single rod progestogen implant and combined oestrogen and progestogen injectables. The copper IUD has been provided significantly less frequently than other contraceptive methods but signs of an increase in most provinces were reported. The most frequently provided method was injectable progesterone, which the article acknowledged was not ideal and emphasised condom use with this method because it can can increase the risk of HIV: The product made up 49% of South Africa's contraceptive use and up to 90% in some provinces.

Tanzanian provider perspectives address the obstacles to consistent contraceptive use in their communities. It was found that the capability of dispensaries to service patients was determined by inconsistent reproductive goals, low educational attainment, misconceptions about the side effects of contraceptives, and social factors such as gender dynamics, spousal dynamics, economic conditions, religious norms, cultural norms, and constraints in supply chains. A provider referenced and example of propaganda spread about the side effects of contraception: "There are influential people, for example elders and religious leaders. They normally convince people that condoms contain some microorganisms and contraceptive pills cause cancer". Another said that women often had pressure from their spouse or family that caused them to use birth control secretly or to discontinue use, and that women frequently preferred undetectable methods for this reason. Access was also hindered as a result of a lack in properly trained medical personnel: "Shortage of the medical attendant...is a challenge, we are not able to attend to a big number of clients, also we do not have enough education which makes us unable to provide women with the methods they want". The majority of medical centers were staffed by people without medical training and few doctors and nurses, despite federal regulations, due to lack of resources. One center had only one person who was able to insert and remove implants, and without her they were unable to service people who wanted an implant inserted or removed. Another dispensary that carried two methods of birth control shared that they sometimes run out of both materials at the same time. Constraints in supply chains sometimes cause dispensaries to run out of contraceptive materials. Providers also claimed that more male involvement and education would be helpful. Public health officials, researchers, and programs can gain a more comprehensive picture of the barriers they face, and the efficacy of current approaches to family planning, by tracking specific, standardized family planning and reproductive health indicators.

Neonatal Nursing

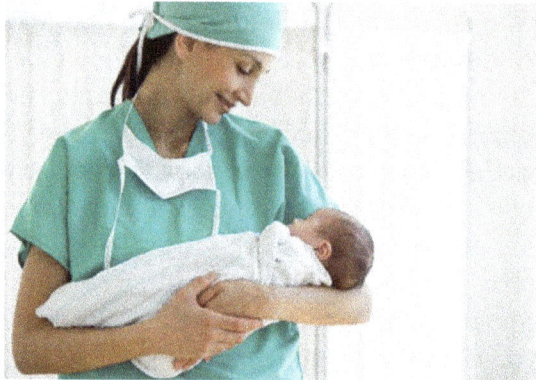

Neonatal nurses (RNs) and neonatal nurse practitioners (NNPs) may work in clinics, community-based settings, hospitals or neonatal intensive care units. They may also conduct research, act as consultants or provide education to staff and family members. This nursing career requires a high level of diligence and teamwork. You will work closely with parents, neonatologists and other nurse specialists to achieve optimal results for your tiny patients.

There are three levels in the neonatal nursing specialty:

- Level I care for healthy infants. The demand for this level of neonatal nursing is decreasing because mothers and newborn babies are now more likely to stay in the same room together after birth.

- Level II nurses are much more in demand because premature and sick babies need constant attention.

- Level III nurses have the most intensive responsibilities, working in the NICU and monitoring seriously ill or premature infants around the clock. They check ventilators and incubators, make sure babies are responding well, and teach parents how to care for their infants properly.

References

- International technical guidance on sexuality education: an evidence-informed approach (PDF). Paris: UNESCO. 2018. p. 22. ISBN 978-92-3-100259-5.

- Reproductive-health: wpro.who.int, Retrieved 14 June 2018

- Department of Health, Republic of South Africa (2014). "Bookshelf: National Contraception and Fertility Planning Policy and Service Delivery Guidelines". Reproductive Health Matters. 22 (43): 200–203. doi:10.1016/S0968-8080(14)43764-9. JSTOR 43288351.

- "Preventing early pregnancy and poor reproductive outcomes among adolescents in developing countries". World Health Organization. Retrieved September 23, 2017.

- Neonatal-nursing: allnursingschools.com, Retrieved 28 May 2018

- Morris JL, Rushwan H (October 2015). "Adolescent sexual and reproductive health: The global challenges". International Journal of Gynaecology and Obstetrics. 131 Suppl 1: S40–2. doi:10.1016/j.ijgo.2015.02.006. PMID 26433504.

Patient Safety and Records

Patient health records help to reduce errors related to prescription drugs, preventive and emergency care, and tests and procedures for ensuring patient safety. Keeping checks for drug-food interactions, allergies, drug dosages, patient information, etc. are all encompassed in patient health records. This chapter includes vital information on patient record maintenance for patient safety and discusses the aspects of medical error, electronic health record, evidence-based medicine, etc.

Patient Safety

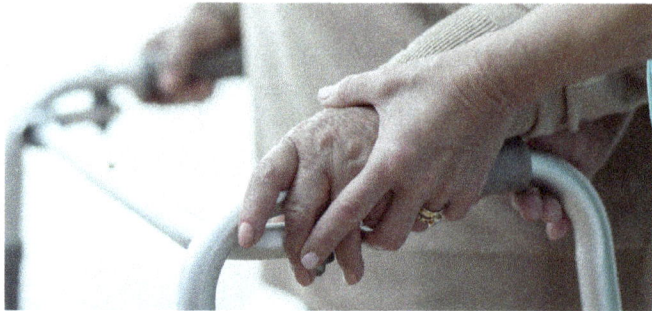

Patient safety is concerned with the way how hospitals and other health care organizations protect their patients from errors, injuries, accidents, and infections.

Patient safety is an issue for all countries that deliver health services, whether they are privately commissioned or funded by the government. Prescribing antibiotics without regard for the patient's underlying condition and whether antibiotics will help the patient, or administering multiple drugs without attention to the potential for adverse drug reactions, all have the potential for harm and patient injury. Patients are not only harmed by the misuse of technology, they can also be harmed by poor communication between different health-care providers or delays in receiving treatment.

Patient safety is a broad subject incorporating the latest technology such as electronic prescribing and redesigning hospitals and services to washing hands correctly and being a team player. Many of the features of patient safety do not involve financial resources; rather, they involve commitment of individuals to practise safely. Individual doctors and nurses can improve patient safety by engaging with patients and their families, checking procedures, learning from errors and communicating effectively with the health-care team. Such activities can also save costs because they minimize the harm caused to patients. When errors are reported and analysed they can help identify the main contributing factors. Understanding the factors that lead to errors is essential for thinking about changes that will prevent errors from being made.

The Why, What, Where, How and Who of Patient Safety

Why does the field of patient safety exist: Patient safety as a discipline began in response to evidence that adverse medical events are widespread and preventable, and as noted above, that there is "too much harm." The goal of the field of patient safety is to minimize adverse events and eliminate preventable harm in health care. Depending on one's use of the term "harm," it is possible to aspire to eliminate all harm in health care.

What is the nature of patient safety Patient safety is a relatively new discipline within the health care professions. Graduate degree programs are currently being introduced in recognition of patient safety as a discipline. It is a subject within heath care quality. However, its methods come largely from disciplines outside medicine, particularly from cognitive psychology, human factors engineering, and organizational management science. That, however, is also true of the biomedical sciences that propelled medicine forward to its current extraordinary capacity to cure illnesses. Their methods came from biology, chemistry, physics, and mathematics, among others. Applying safety sciences to health care requires inclusion of experts with new source disciplines, such as engineering, but without any divergence from the goals or inherent nature of the medical profession.

Patient safety is a property that emerges from systems design: Patient safety must be an attribute of the health care system. Patient safety seeks high reliability under conditions of risk. Illness presents the first condition of risk in health care. Patient safety applies to the second condition: the therapeutic intervention. Sometimes the therapeutic risk is audacious, such as when a patient's heart is lifted, chilled, cut, and sewn during cardiac transplantation surgery. Risk and safety are flip sides of the therapeutic coin.

Patient safety demands design of systems to make risky interventions reliable. Two tenets of complexity theory apply: First, the greater the complexity of the system, the greater is the propensity for chaos. Second, in open, interacting systems, unpredictable events will happen. The better the therapeutic design, the more resilient it is in the face of both predictable and unpredictable possible or impending failures, so they can be prevented or rescue can be achieved. Safety systems include design of materials, procedures, environment, training, and the nature of the culture among people operating in the system.

Berwick and others have collaborated with Amalberti to apply Shewhart's notion of statistical quality or error levels to health care. Systems are categorized by their level of adverse events. Barriers to progression from one level to another are identified. Interestingly, leaders of high reliability organizations in other industries view the level of adverse events in medicine as so high that many of them would consider the health industry as existing in a state of chaos. The patient safety discipline seeks systems that can move health care to higher and higher levels of safe care.

Berwick and others have collaborated with Amalberti to apply Shewhart's notion of statistical quality or error levels to health care. Systems are categorized by their level of adverse events. Barriers to progression from one level to another are identified. Interestingly, leaders of high reliability organizations in other industries view the level of adverse events in medicine as so high that many of them would consider the health industry as existing in a state of chaos. The patient safety discipline seeks systems that can move health care to higher and higher levels of safe care.

Patient safety is a property that is designed for the nature of illness. High-reliability design is a concept that was not originally developed for health care. However, health care has some essential features in common with how high-reliability design has evolved. While often complex and unpredictable, it can have the ultimate high-stakes outcome: preservation of life.

A unique feature of patient care is its highly personal nature. Provision of care almost always requires health care workers to cross significant personal boundaries, both psychological and physical. To protect patient integrity, the health professions have developed codes of professional ethics that guide how best to provide health care without doing dishonour to the ill person. Patient safety designs must allow for these important restrictions, which include confidentiality, physical privacy, and others. At times, these needs conflict directly with the transparency and vigilance needed for optimal patient care, including safety.

Another unique feature is the natural progression of illness. By definition, when illness care begins, something has already gone wrong. Thus, in many medical situations, failure to provide the correct intervention causes harm to the patient. A missed diagnosis of meningococcal meningitis, for example, usually results in patient death. The patient safety discipline acknowledges the need to include harm due to omission of action, as well as the obvious harm due to actions taken.

The vast diversity of possible etiologies and manifestations of illness makes systems design in health care a unique challenge. Nonetheless, the reality is that most conditions are common and of common etiology, which allows for optimal design, if not infallible outcomes. If most patients with a condition such as breast cancer are best treated according to protocol but some require offprotocol, tailored treatment, systems can be designed to meet that need for the majority of protocols with tailoring options.

Patient safety is a property dependent on open learning. Patient safety has another inherent feature that derives directly from its dependence on errors and adverse events as a main source of understanding. It depends on a culture of openness to all relevant perspectives in which those involved in adverse events are treated as partners in learning. In this sense, patient safety espouses continuous cycles of learning, reporting of adverse events or near misses, dissemination of lessons learned, and the establishment of cultures that are trusted to not cast unfair blame. The patient safety field marries principles of adult education and effective behavioral learning with the traditional approaches of the medical profession. Known from its early days as the field that seeks to move "beyond blame" to a culture trusted by all to be just patient safety, patient safety pioneers have pushed for a much deeper understanding of the mechanisms of errors that often lie beyond the actions or control of the individual.

Patient safety advocates turn away from the traditions of the guild in which social standing and privileged knowledge shielded practitioners from accountability. They also reject the defensive posture of old risk management approaches in which physicians and leaders of health care organizations were advised to admit no responsibility and to defend all malpractice claims, whether or not they were justified. Patient safety embraces organizational and personal accountability, but it also recognizes the importance of moving beyond blame in both its organizational and its personal dimensions, while maintaining accountability and integrity in interactions with patients and families who have suffered avoidable adverse events.

Trustworthiness is essential to the concept of patient safety. The health care system designed for patient safety is trustworthy. This is not because errors will not be made and adverse events will never happen, but because the health care system holds itself accountable to applying safety sciences optimally. Patient safety (as an attribute) prevents avoidable adverse events by paying attention (as a discipline) to systems and interactions, including human interactions, and allowing learning by all parties from near misses and actual adverse events. Through a concerted, conscientious effort, all those involved act to minimize the extent and impact of unavoidable adverse events by creating well-designed systems and well-motivated, informed, conscientious, and vigilant personnel, and by seeking to repair damage honestly and respectfully when it occurs.

Where does patient safety happen? The ultimate locus of patient safety is the microsystem. That is, the immediate environment in which care occurs—the operating room, the emergency department, and so on. It is in the microsystem where the "sharp end" resides, where patient care giver interactions occur, where failures of safety emerge, and where patients are harmed. Breaches in safety may have occurred in many blunt-end components, events constitute properties of interacting components of the overall system. Therefore, patient safety is irreducibly a matter of systems. Nonetheless, as the setting where the patient receives health care, the microsystem is the locus where the successes or failures of all systems to ensure safety converge.

At the same time, patient safety must be concerned with the entire system. Importantly, patient safety recognizes that the microsystem is inherently unpredictable. Although it takes a mechanistic view of causation, patient safety acknowledges that each microsystem is open in that it can be influenced by another microsystem. This may result in something unpredictable. Thus, for instance, the microsystem of concern in surgical safety might be the operating suite, but if a local emergency demands that two members of the surgical team leave the operating room, the microsystem has been unpredictably affected.

Ways through which Patient Safety is Achieved

A number of mechanisms are involved in achieving patient safety.

High-reliability design: The fundamental mechanism by which patient safety can be achieved is high-reliability design, which includes many components. Thus, the irreducible unit of patient safety delivery is multifaceted; all components of health care delivery must be integrated into a system that is as reliable as possible under complex conditions.

A unique feature of high-reliability design comes from complexity theory, which notes that open, interacting systems will produce some level of chaos or inherently unpredictable events. High reliability designs are resilient even when unpredictable events occur.

Additional design features that guide health systems engineers include "lean process" and a notion of breaking through reliability boundaries in leaps from one safety level to another. These 9 levels of reliability are often known as sigma levels—through the use of simplified and better processes.

The concept of a multi-layered system, in which the failures within each of the layers must be aligned for an error to occur, is known as the "Swiss cheese" model of accident causation. The components that make up the system include the institution and its organization, the professional team and the individuals it includes, and the technology in use.

Error traps (i.e., unpredictable situations in which error is highly likely) are another vivid concept on which safety sciences focus. The notion is that health care delivery is not only complex; it is also an open interacting system, in which illness is also a given, so the opportunities for making errors are many and endemic. Health care workers and health systems designers must therefore take this into account.

Safety systems design in health care is early in its development. Practical approaches to design for safety have been pioneered by the Institute for Healthcare Improvement (IHI), the Agency for Healthcare Research and Quality (AHRQ), and the World Health Organization's (WHO) World Alliance for Patient Safety, among others. For instance, patient safety designs can be thought of as falling into two types: those that are for types of routine care that vary little and can best be managed with protocols allowing for little deviation, and those that are for unique situations where on-the-spot innovation and significant deviation from protocol are required.

Patient Advocacy

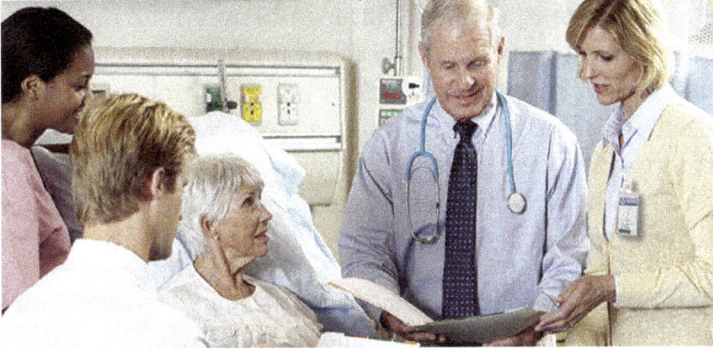

An advocate is one who pleads the cause of another; and a patient advocate is an advocate for clients' rights. In that role, the nurse protects the client's human and legal rights and provides assistance in asserting those rights if the need arises. Advocacy may include, for example, providing additional information for a patient who is trying to decide whether or not to accept a treatment. Or, the nurse may defend a patient's rights in a general way by speaking out against policies or action that might endanger their well-being or conflict with their rights.

There are several steps involved in being an effective patient advocate:

1. Make sure the client agrees to receiving the information.

2. Either have the necessary information or know how to get it.

3. Want the client to have the information.

4. Present the information in a way that is meaningful to the client.

5. Accept the fact that there may be those who do not wish the client to be informed.

An advocate must know how to provide support in an objective manner. They must be careful not to convey approval or disapproval of the client's choices. Underlying patient advocacy are the beliefs that individual have the following rights:

• The right to select values they deem necessary to sustain their lives.

• The right to decide which course of action will best achieve the chosen values.

• The right to dispose of values in any way they choose without coercion by others.

Barriers to Nursing Advocacy

When we talk about coercion by others or those who do not wish the client to be informed we are talking to about just some of the barriers nurses can face when advocating for their patients. By analyzing the barriers to effective advocacy nurses can then develop strategies to manage those obstacles and maximize their advocacy efforts.

The most common attribute is conflict of interest between the nurse's responsibility to the patient and the nurse's duty to the institution where the nurse is employed. Other barriers include lack of support and lack of power. Threats of punishment are also considered an attribute of barriers to nursing advocacy, like being reprimanded, poor evaluations, and ultimately being fired. Finally, a historical barrier of nursing being a feminine profession with a tradition of subservience to the medical profession is also considered a barrier to nursing advocacy.

The implications for nursing practice are that nurses need to overcome barriers to become effective nursing advocates for their clients. That would be in an ideal situation however, the threat of job loss, retribution, intimidation, or ostracism are very real. Nurses need strategies to overcome barriers so that they can provide the best possible education and services for their patients.

Strategies for Overcoming Barriers

The biggest barrier most nurses face when acting as a patient advocate are institutional barriers. Every nurse must know the definition of their scope of practice in both their practice state, and their healthcare facility. How the nurse's role is defined is different behind every door. Nurses may find little to no support in the advocacy role from administrators, physicians, and even nursing peers. Knowing the written rules will help be a more effective advocate.

Clear, effective communication will help overcome institutional barriers when in advocate mode. The nurse's ideas and suggestions will be better received if spoken clearly and emotional reactions like anger and frustration are kept to a minimum. Body language counts. Every OR nurse knows even with the face almost completely covered the eyes can give away every secret. Leaning forward, pointing fingers, or crossing arms across the chest can all be viewed as hostile or confrontational.

Language, both spoken and written, makes a difference in the effectiveness of client advocacy, as well. Keep the focus on the patient. Document everything. If you have an interaction with the patient and they express a strong opinion, for or against a treatment option or plan of care, make sure you put it in your nurse's notes and put a copy on the front of the chart for all to see or make a point of discussing with a nurse manager or the physician so everyone is aware of the patient's concerns.

Knowing where your professional organizations stand on the subject of advocacy can also be helpful but don't count on that holding any real weight if a conflict arises. Learn your employer's administrative structure, what committees might support your advocacy track and talk to your peers; they may have dealt with similar situations and be able to provide practical advice.

Navigating the complex world of hospitals and medical treatment can be challenging under the best of circumstances. When someone is seriously ill, the situation can become even more difficult. For this reason, some people choose to hire a professional patient advocate to speak on their behalf and help guide them through the decisions involved in treating whatever condition they may be suffering from. If you have a loved one who has been hospitalized, you can fulfil this role yourself. If you are a well-organized, assertive, and caring person, you can help a friend or family member as their advocate.

Collecting Information for the Patient

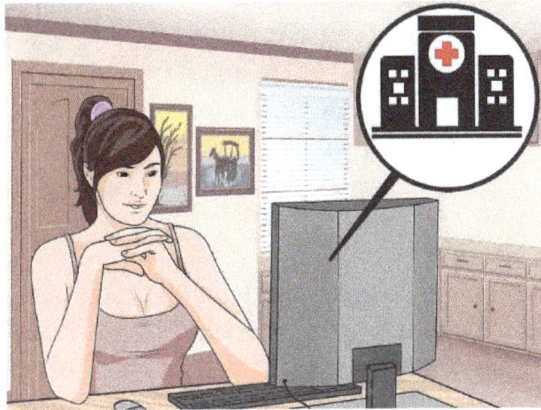

1. Do some background research: The more familiar you are with the health care system, the insurance system, and the specific medical condition your loved one is grappling with, the more effective you can be as an advocate.

- For example, take some time to learn how the hospital bureaucracy works. What is the "chain of command?" Who does your loved-one's doctor or medical team report to?

- Learn about the patient's health insurance policy and/or Medicare aid. Look into the process of appealing when aid is denied.

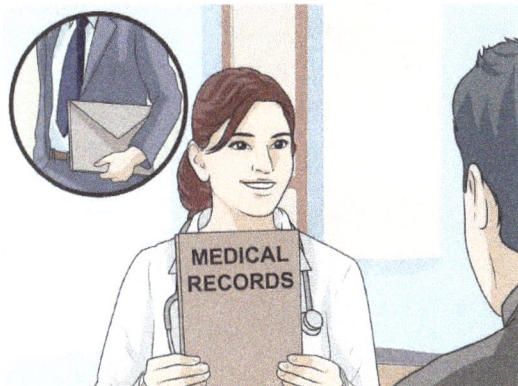

2 Collect the patient's medical documents. Gather all relevant documents related to your loved-one's hospitalization and treatment. This might include test results, explanations of benefits, bills, and prescriptions.

- Keep all these records in one place and organized in such a way that you can find whatever you might need to reference later. Keep the same types of documents together, and organize them by date.

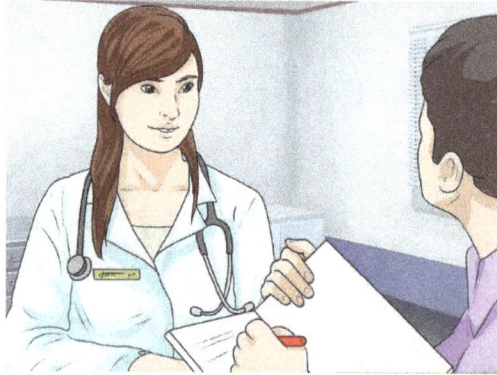

3. Take notes. Keep a journal or notepad handy at all times. Make notes every time you talk to the doctor or other health care professionals. These sessions can be very brief, but contain a lot of information, so keeping track of it all for later later reference can be helpful.

- Make note of who you've spoken to and what everyone says. Your loved one may be seen by several different doctors and nurses. Record all their names. This will make it much easier to have conversations later about the recommendations or information provided by each physician.

- Make sure to note the date of every conversation as well. Then if you have a question about something you've been told, you can be specific, i.e. "Last Wednesday you told me X, but now you're telling me Y instead. What has changed since last time we spoke?"

Communicating with and on Behalf of the Patient

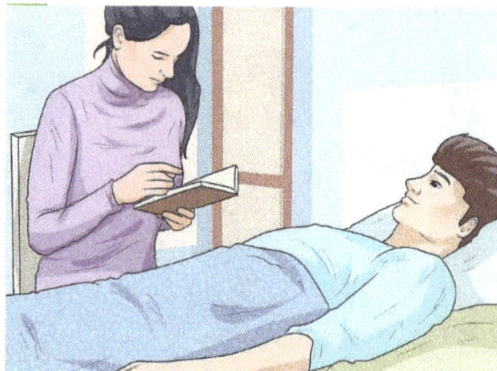

1 Help keep the patient grounded. Long hospital stays can be disorienting and con-fusing, especially for the elderly. Talk and read to the patient in calm, soothing tones. Answer their questions in a clear but reassuring manner.

- Long hospital stays can promote the onset of delirium, a severe state of disori-entation or confusion that can make it difficult for someone to think, rest, or follow directions. This condition may be made more likely by certain drugs that may be used to relieve pain, such as narcotics (analgesics) and sedative hypnot-ics (benzodiazepines). If you suspect the onset of delirium, contact hospital staff and ask what assistance they can provide.

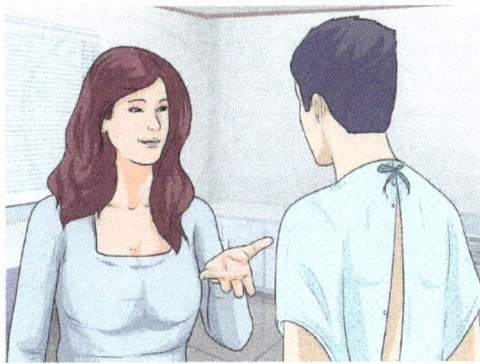

2 Present information and options to the patient. One job of the advocate is to act as an intermediary between the doctor and the patient. Chances are, you will end up col-lecting a lot of very complex information about the patient's condition and treatment options. Help clarify the information and treatment options.

- Keep in mind that this situation may be very overwhelming for the patient, and there is a lot to keep track of. Don't talk down to the patient, but do present things in as straightforward a manner as possible.

- Avoid medical jargon and other technical language when possible.

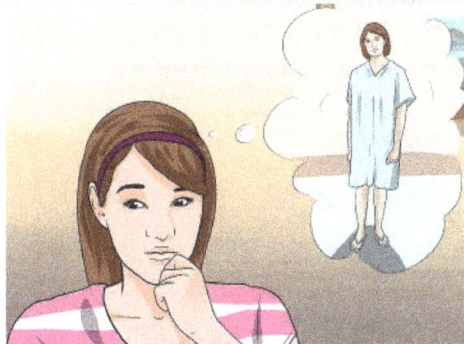

3 Find out what the patient wants. Make sure you know what the patient wants, both from you and in terms of treatment. You can only be an effective advocate if you have

a clear understanding of your loved one's desires. This conversation is best had before the person is severely ill. It is everyone's best interest to invest time and energy into living wills, assigning power of attorney, and advance directives so family and loved ones do not have to grasp at straws when faced with a health tragedy.

- Depending on the severity of the health issue, the patient may or may not feel up to communicating their desires to doctors and other medical staff.

- Part of this process may involve helping the patient weigh their options to make the best decision for treatment. Being familiar with the patient's values and belief systems can be important, especially if his or her condition is life-threatening.

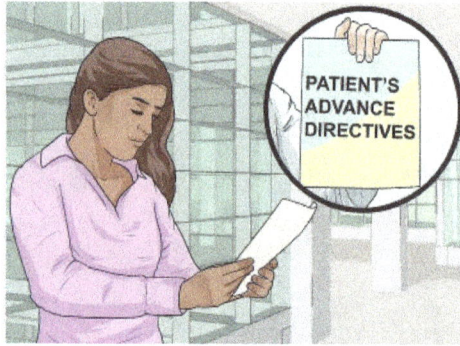

4 Look into advance directives. It is a good idea to find out if the patient has an advance directive. This is a document that provides the hospital with instructions as to what should be done if they become incapable of expressing their desires.

- This might include specific instructions, such as a desire not be put on life support if brain death occurs. Or, it may include instructions to designate a certain person as responsible for making decisions on the patient's behalf (a proxy directive, also called "durable power of attorney"). Ideally, if there is a proxy directive, it should designate you, the advocate, as the patient's proxy.

If the patient does not have an advance directive, it may be a good idea to encourage them to complete one, and to help the patient through this process. The paperwork for an advance directive varies from one state to the next.

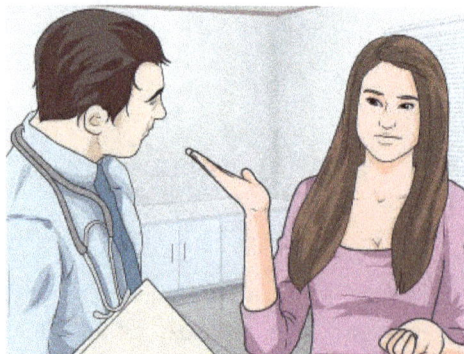

5 Communicate the patient's questions and concerns to the doctor. It is your responsibility to ensure that any questions or concerns the patient has are conveyed to the doctor. This is especially true if they feel incapable of or reluctant about asking questions.

- Ask for clarification when necessary. Doctors and hospitals, for example, use a lot of acronyms. If a doctor is talking in jargon you don't understand, ask them to explain things in simpler language.

- If you are a non-family member, the patient will need to sign some paperwork so that healthcare workers can share information with you. Ask about release of information paperwork so that you can legally be informed about the patient's treatment.

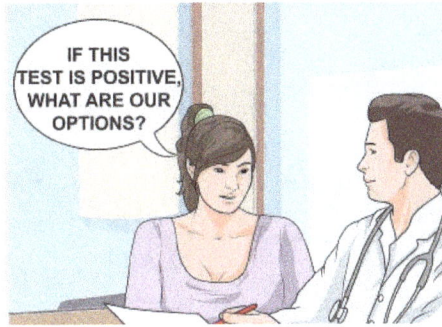

6 Speak assertively on the patient's behalf. Your most important role as advocate is to make sure the doctor and other hospital staff understand and follow the patient's wishes. This will require you to be clear and politely assertive.

- Use plain language to tell the doctor what the patient's desires are.

- Ask questions about follow up treatments, next steps, and what will happen as a result of different test outcomes. For example: "if this test is positive, what are our options?"

- Get a second opinion if necessary. If your loved one wants a second opinion, or what the doctor is telling you doesn't seem right based on the information you've gathered, be direct about asking for and seeking a second opinion.

Making Life Easier for the Patient

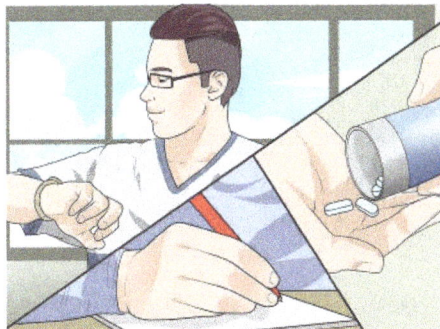

1 Help with medication regimens. For serious health conditions, the number of medications a patient must sometimes take can be overwhelming. As an advocate, you can help your loved one by keeping a list of which medications they are taking.

- Make note of which medications should be taken at what time. Provide reminders or any other assistance the patient may ask for to ensure medications are taken on schedule.

- Use a medication planner with time slots designated for dosing schedules. There are daily medication planners and multi-time slot medication planners to make this more successful if the patient has multiple doses of medication throughout the day. You can also look into different medication reminder apps for your smartphone.

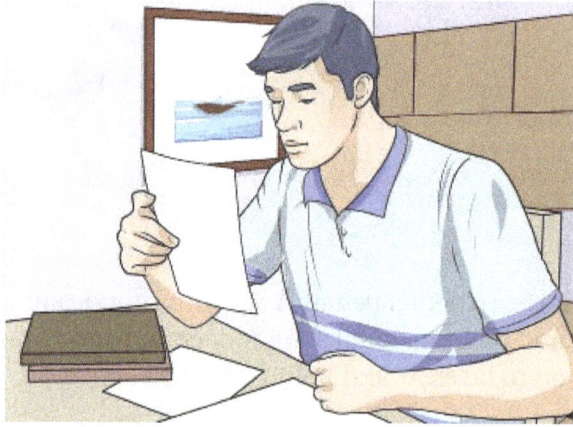

2 Do the paperwork. You can also help your loved one by taking care of necessary paperwork for them. This will be one less thing weighing on their mind during this stressful time.

- This could include forms and paperwork from the hospital itself, as well as insurance documents and applications for employer-provided benefits.

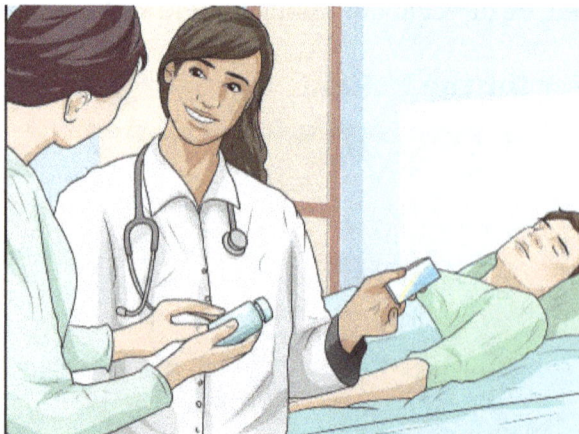

3 Watch for errors. Hospitals can be chaotic places, and errors by doctors, nurses and other staff are common. This problem is especially pronounced in the administration of medication.

Make sure your loved one is receiving the correct medication in the correct dose, and that they do not have an allergy to anything the doctor has prescribed.

The nurse should verify the medication, allergies and time of dose with the patient to avoid and mistakes. Nursing staff observe the five rights of medication administration — right patient, right dose, right drug, right time, and right route.

Take special note of any new medications, and ask questions about how long and when the medication should be taken, as well as what side effects it might cause.

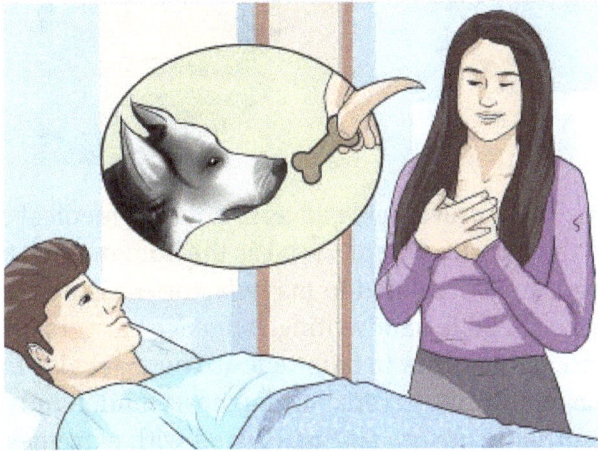

4 Provide other services as needed. An advocate is often asked to take on a variety of other tasks. This could be anything from transportation to caring for pets.

- Take on any task that the patient asks you to and that you are comfortable and capable of carrying out. Ask regularly what you can do to help. There may be many ways you can provide help that you haven't thought of yet.

Patient Abuse

Patient abuse or neglect is any action or failure to act which causes unreasonable suffering, misery or harm to the patient.

- Abuse includes physically striking or sexually assaulting a patient. It also includes the intentional withholding of necessary food, physical care, and medical attention.

- Neglect includes the failure to properly attend to the needs and care of a patient, or the unintentional causing of injury to a patient, whether by act or omission.

Patient abuse and neglect may occur in settings such as hospitals, nursing homes, clinics and during home-based care.

Medical Error

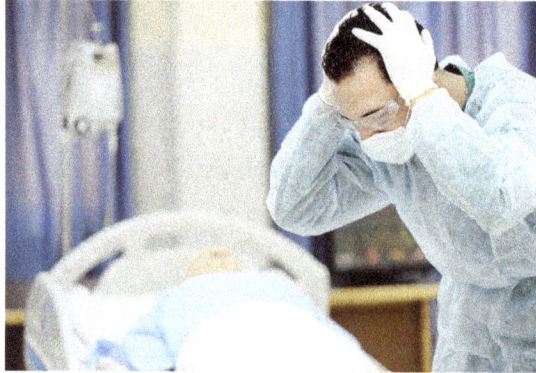

Medical error is defined as a preventable adverse effect of medical care whether or not evident or harmful to the patient. Often viewed as the human error factor in healthcare, this is a highly complex subject related to many factors such as incompetency, lack of education or experience, illegible handwriting, language barriers, inaccurate documentation, gross negligence, and fatigue to name a few. There are also many different types of errors ranging from medication errors, misdiagnosis, under and over treatment, and surgical mishaps. Medical errors are also associated with extremes of age, new procedures, urgency, and the severity of the medical condition being treated.

The subject of medical errors is not a new one. However, it did not come to widespread attention in the until the 1990s, when government-sponsored research about the problem was undertaken by two physicians, Lucian Leape and David Bates. In 1999, a report compiled by the Committee on Quality of Health Care in America and published by the Institute of Medicine (IOM) made headlines with its findings. As a result of the IOM report, President Clinton asked the Quality Interagency Coordination Task Force (QuIC) to analyze the problem of medical errors and patient safety, and make recommendations for improvement. The Report to the President on Medical Errors was published in February 2000.

It is important to understand the terms used by the government and health care professionals in describing medical errors in order to distinguish between injury or death resulting from mistakes made by people on the one hand, and unfortunate results of treatment on the other. Some allergic reactions to medications or failures to respond to cancer treatment, for example, result from physical differences among patients or the known side effects of certain treatments, and not from prescribing the wrong drug or therapy for the patient's condition. This type of negative outcome is called an adverse event in official documents. Adverse events can be defined as undesirable and unintentional, though not necessarily unexpected, results of medical treatment. An example of an adverse event is discomfort in an artificial joint that continues after the expected recovery period, or a chronic headache following a spinal tap.

A medical error, on the other hand, is an adverse event that could be prevented given the current state of medical knowledge. The QuIC task force expanded the IOM's working definition of a medical error to cover as many types of mistakes as possible. Their definition of a medical error is as follows: "The failure of a planned action to be completed as intended or the use of a wrong plan to achieve an aim. Errors can include problems in practice, products, procedures, and systems." The National Patient Safety Foundation (NPSF) prefers the term "healthcare error" to "medical error," and defines such errors as follows: "An unintended healthcare outcome caused by a defect in the delivery of care to a patient. Healthcare errors may be errors of commission (doing the wrong thing), omission (not doing the right thing), or execution (doing the right thing incorrectly)." A useful brief definition of a medical error is that it is a preventable adverse event.

Causes

Medical errors are associated with inexperienced physicians and nurses, new procedures, extremes of age, and complex or urgent care. Poor communication (whether in one's own language or, as may be the case for medical tourists, another language), improper documentation, illegible handwriting, spelling errors, inadequate nurse-to-patient ratios, and similarly named medications are also known to contribute to the problem. Patient actions may also contribute significantly to medical errors. Falls, for example, may result from patients' own misjudgements. Human error has been implicated in nearly 80 percent of adverse events that occur in complex healthcare systems. The vast majority of medical errors result from faulty systems and poorly designed processes versus poor practices or incompetent practitioners.

Healthcare Complexity

Complicated technologies, powerful drugs, intensive care, and prolonged hospital stay can contribute to medical errors.

System and Process Design

In 2000, The Institute of Medicine released "To Err is Human," which asserted that the problem in medical errors is not bad people in health care it is that good people are working in bad systems that need to be made safer.

Poor communication and unclear lines of authority of physicians, nurses, and other care providers are also contributing factors. Disconnected reporting systems within a hospital can result in fragmented systems in which numerous hand-offs of patients results in lack of coordination and errors.

Other factors include the impression that action is being taken by other groups within the institution, reliance on automated systems to prevent error., and inadequate systems to share information about errors, which hampers analysis of contributory causes and improvement strategies. Cost-cutting measures by hospitals in response to reimbursement cutbacks can compromise patient safety. In emergencies, patient care may be rendered in areas poorly suited for safe monitoring. The American Institute of Architects has identified concerns for the safe design and construction of health care facilities. Infrastructure failure is also a concern. According to the WHO, 50% of medical equipment in developing countries is only partly usable due to lack of skilled operators or parts. As a result, diagnostic procedures or treatments cannot be performed, leading to substandard treatment.

The Joint Commission's Annual Report on Quality and Safety 2007 found that inadequate communication between healthcare providers, or between providers and the patient and family members, was the root cause of over half the serious adverse events in accredited hospitals. Other leading causes included inadequate assessment of the patient's condition, and poor leadership or training.

Competency, Education and Training

Variations in healthcare provider training & experience and failure to acknowledge the prevalence and seriousness of medical errors also increase the risk. The so-called July effect occurs when new residents arrive at teaching hospitals, causing an increase in medication errors according to a study of data from 1979-2006.

Human Factors and Ergonomics

Cognitive errors commonly encountered in medicine were initially identified by psychologists Amos Tversky and Daniel Kahneman in the early 1970s. Jerome Groopman, author of *How Doctors Think*, says these are "cognitive pitfalls", biases which cloud our logic. For example, a practitioner may overvalue the first data encountered, skewing his thinking (or recent or dramatic cases which come quickly to mind and may color judgement). Another pitfall is where stereotypes may prejudice thinking.

Sleep deprivation has also been cited as a contributing factor in medical errors. One study found that being awake for over 24 hours caused medical interns to double or triple the number of preventable medical errors, including those that resulted in injury or death. The risk of car crash after these shifts increased by 168%, and the risk of near miss by 460%. Interns admitted falling asleep during lectures, during rounds, and even during surgeries. Night shifts are associated with worse surgeon performance during laparoscopic surgeries.

Practitioner risk factors include fatigue, depression, and burnout. Factors related to the clinical setting include diverse patients, unfamiliar settings, time pressures, and increased patient-to-nurse staffing ratio increases. Drug names that look alike or sound alike are also a problem.

Examples

Errors can include misdiagnosis or delayed diagnosis, administration of the wrong drug to the wrong patient or in the wrong way, giving multiple drugs that interact negatively, surgery on an incorrect site, failure to remove all surgical instruments, failure to take the correct blood type into account, or incorrect record-keeping. A 10th type of error is ones which are not watched for by researchers, such as RNs failing to program an IV pump to give a full dose of IV antibiotics or other medication.

Errors in Diagnosis

A large study reported several cases where patients were wrongly told that they were HIV-negative when the physicians erroneously ordered and interpreted HTLV (a closely related virus) testing rather than HIV testing. In the same study, >90% of HTLV tests were ordered erroneously. It is estimated that between 10-15 percent of physician diagnoses are erroneous.

Misdiagnosis of lower extremity cellulitis is estimated to occur in 30% of patients, leading to unnecessary hospitalizations in 85% and unnecessary antibiotic use in 92%. Collectively, these errors lead to between 50,000 and 130,000 unnecessary hospitalizations and between $195 and $515 million in avoidable health care spending annually in the United States.

Misdiagnosis of Psychological Disorders

Female sexual desire sometimes used to be diagnosed as female hysteria.

Sensitivities to foods and food allergies risk being misdiagnosed as the anxiety disorder Orthorexia.

Studies have found that bipolar disorder has often been misdiagnosed as major depression. Its early diagnosis necessitates that clinicians pay attention to the features of the patient's depression and also look for present or prior hypomanic or manic symptomatology.

The misdiagnosis of schizophrenia is also a common problem. There may be long delays of patients getting a correct diagnosis of this disorder.

The DSM-5 field trials included "test-retest reliability" which involved different clinicians doing independent evaluations of the same patient—a new approach to the study of diagnostic reliability.

Outpatient vs. Inpatient

Misdiagnosis is the leading cause of medical error in outpatient facilities. Since the National Institute of Medicine's 1999 report, "To Err is Human," found up to 98,000 hospital patients die from preventable medical errors in the U.S. each year, government and private sector efforts have focused on inpatient safety.

After an Error has Occurred

Mistakes can have a strongly negative emotional impact on the doctors who commit them.

Recognizing that Mistakes are not Isolated Events

Some physicians recognize that adverse outcomes from errors usually do not happen because of an isolated error and actually reflect system problems. This concept is often referred to as the Swiss Cheese model. This is the concept that there are layers of protection for clinicians and patients to prevent mistakes from occurring. Therefore, even if a doctor or nurse makes a small error (e.g. incorrect dose of drug written on a drug chart by doctor), this is picked up before it actually affects patient care (e.g. pharmacist checks the drug chart and rectifies the error). Such mechanisms include: Practical alterations (e.g.-medications that cannot be given through IV, are fitted with tubing which means they cannot be linked to an IV even if a clinician makes a mistake and tries to), systematic safety processes (e.g. all patients must have a Waterlow score assessment and falls assessment completed on admission), and training programmes/continuing professional development courses are measures that may be put in place.

There may be several breakdowns in processes to allow one adverse outcome. In addition, errors are more common when other demands compete for a physician's attention. However, placing too much blame on the system may not be constructive.

Placing the Practice of Medicine in Perspective

Essayists imply that the potential to make mistakes is part of what makes being a physician rewarding and without this potential the rewards of medical practice would be diminished. Laurence states that "Everybody dies, you and all of your patients. All relationships end. Would you want it any other way? [...] Don't take it personally" Seder states "[...] if I left medicine, I would mourn its loss as I've mourned the passage of my poetry. On a daily basis, it is both a privilege and a joy to have the trust of patients and their families and the camaraderie of peers. There is no challenge to make your blood race like that of a difficult case, no mind game as rigorous as the challenging differential diagnosis, and though the stakes are high, so are the rewards."

Disclosing Mistakes

Forgiveness, which is part of many cultural traditions, may be important in coping with medical mistakes.

To Oneself

Inability to forgive oneself may create a cycle of distress and increased likelihood of a future error.

However, Wu et al. suggest "...those who coped by accepting responsibility were more likely to make constructive changes in practice, but [also] to experience more emotional distress." It may be helpful to consider the much larger number of patients who are not exposed to mistakes and are helped by medical care.

To Patients

Gallagher et al. state that patients want "information about what happened, why the error happened, how the error's consequences will be mitigated, and how recurrences will be prevented." Interviews with patients and families reported in a 2003 book by Rosemary Gibson and Janardan Prasad Singh, put forward that those who have been harmed by medical errors face a "wall of silence" and "want an acknowledgement" of the harm. With honesty, "healing can begin not just for the patients and their families but also the doctors, nurses and others involved." Detailed suggestions on how to disclose are available.

A 2005 study by Wendy Levinson of the University of Toronto showed surgeons discussing medical errors used the word "error" or "mistake" in only 57 percent of disclosure conversations and offered a verbal apology only 47 percent of the time.

Patient disclosure is important in the medical error process. The current standard of practice at many hospitals is to disclose errors to patients when they occur. In the past, it was a common fear that disclosure to the patient would incite a malpractice lawsuit. Many physicians would not explain that an error had taken place, causing a lack of trust toward the healthcare community. In 2007, 34 states passed legislation that precludes any information from a physician's apology for a medical error from being used in malpractice court (even a full admission of fault). This encourages physicians to acknowledge and explain mistakes to patients, keeping an open line of communication.

The American Medical Association's Council on Ethical and Judicial Affairs states in its ethics code:

> "Situations occasionally occur in which a patient suffers significant medical complications that may have resulted from the physician's mistake or judgment.

In these situations, the physician is ethically required to inform the patient of all facts necessary to ensure understanding of what has occurred. Concern regarding legal liability which might result following truthful disclosure should not affect the physician's honesty with a patient."

From the American College of Physicians Ethics Manual:

"In addition, physicians should disclose to patients information about procedural or judgment errors made in the course of care if such information is material to the patient's well-being. Errors do not necessarily constitute improper, negligent, or unethical behavior, but failure to disclose them may."

However, "there appears to be a gap between physicians' attitudes and practices regarding error disclosure. Willingness to disclose errors was associated with higher training level and a variety of patient-centered attitudes, and it was not lessened by previous exposure to malpractice litigation". Hospital administrators may share these concerns.

Consequently, in the United States, many states have enacted laws excluding expressions of sympathy after accidents as proof of liability. However, "excluding from admissibility in court proceedings apologetic expressions of sympathy but not fault-admitting apologies after accidents".

Disclosure may actually reduce malpractice payments.

To Non-physicians

In a study of physicians who reported having made a mistake, it was offered that disclosing to non-physician sources of support may reduce stress more than disclosing to physician colleagues. This may be due to the finding that of the physicians in the same study, when presented with a hypothetical scenario of a mistake made by another colleague, only 32% of them would have unconditionally offered support. It is possible that greater benefit occurs when spouses are physicians.

To Other Physicians

Discussing mistakes with other physicians is beneficial. However, medical providers may be less forgiving of one another. The reason is not clear, but one essayist has admonished, "don't take too much joy in the mistakes of other doctors."

To the Physician's Institution

Disclosure of errors, especially 'near misses' may be able to reduce subsequent errors in institutions that are capable of reviewing near misses. However, doctors report that institutions may not be supportive of the doctor.

Use of Rationalization to Cover up Medical Errors

Based on anecdotal and survey evidence, Banja states that rationalization (making excuses) is very common among the medical profession to cover up medical errors.

By Presence of to the Patient

A survey of more than 10,000 physicians in the United States came to the results that, on the question "Are there times when it's acceptable to cover up or avoid revealing a mistake if that mistake would not cause harm to the patient?", 19% answered yes, 60% answered no and 21% answered it depends. On the question "Are there times when it is acceptable to cover up or avoid revealing a mistake if that mistake would potentially or likely harm the patient?", 2% answered yes, 95% answered no and 3% answered it depends.

Cause-specific Preventive Measures

Traditionally, errors are attributed to mistakes made by individuals who may be penalized for these mistakes. The usual approach to correct the errors is to create new rules with additional checking steps in the system, aiming to prevent further errors. As an example, an error of free flow IV administration of heparin is approached by teaching staff how to use the IV systems and to use special care in setting the IV pump. While overall errors become less likely, the checks add to workload and may in themselves be a cause of additional errors.

A newer model for improvement in medical care takes its origin from the work of W. Edwards Deming in a model of Total Quality Management. In this model, there is an attempt to identify the underlying system defect that allowed the opportunity for the error to occur. As an example, in such a system the error of free flow IV administration of Heparin is dealt with by not using IV heparin and substituting subcutaneous administration of heparin, obviating the entire problem. However, such an approach presupposes available research showing that subcutaneous heparin is as effective as IV. Thus, most systems use a combination of approaches to the problem.

In Specific Specialties

The field of medicine that has taken the lead in systems approaches to safety is anaesthesiology. Steps such as standardization of IV medications to 1 ml doses, national and international color-coding standards, and development of improved airway support devices has made anesthesia care a model of systems improvement in care.

Pharmacy professionals have extensively studied the causes of errors in the prescribing, preparation, dispensing and administration of medications. As far back as the 1930s, pharmacists worked with physicians to select, from many options, the safest and most effective drugs available for use in hospitals. The process is known as the

Formulary System and the list of drugs is known as the Formulary. In the 1960s, hospitals implemented unit dose packaging and unit dose drug distribution systems to reduce the risk of wrong drug and wrong dose errors in hospitalized patients; centralized sterile admixture services were shown to decrease the risks of contaminated and infected intravenous medications; and pharmacists provided drug information and clinical decision support directly to physicians to improve the safe and effective use of medications. Pharmacists are recognized experts in medication safety and have made many contributions that reduce error and improve patient care over the last 50 years. More recently, governments have attempted to address issues like patient-pharmacists communication and consumer knowledge through measures like the Australian Government's Quality Use of Medicines policy.

Prevention

Medical care is frequently compared adversely to aviation; while many of the factors that lead to errors in both fields are similar, aviation's error management protocols are regarded as much more effective. Safety measures include informed consent, the availability of a second practitioner's opinion, voluntary reporting of errors, root cause analysis, reminders to improve patient medication adherence, hospital accreditation, and systems to ensure review by experienced or specialist practitioners.

A template has been developed for the design (both structure and operation) of hospital medication safety programmes, particularly for acute tertiary settings, which emphasizes safety culture, infrastructure, data (error detection and analysis), communication and training.

Particularly to prevent the medication errors in the perspective of the intrathecal administration of local anaesthetics, there is a proposal to change the presentation and packaging of the appliances and agents used for this purpose. One spinal needle with a syringe prefilled with the local anaesthetic agents may be marketed in a single blister pack, which will be peeled open and presented before the anaesthesiologist conducting the procedure.

Reporting Requirements

In the United States, adverse medical event reporting systems were mandated in just over half (27) of the states as of 2014, a figure unchanged since 2007. In U.S. hospitals error reporting is a condition of payment by Medicare. An investigation by the Office of Inspector General, Department of Health and Human Services released January 6, 2012 found that most errors are not reported and even in the case of errors that are reported and investigated changes are seldom made which would prevent them in the future. The investigation revealed that there was often lack of knowledge regarding which events were reportable and recommended that lists of reportable events be developed.

Misconceptions

These are the common misconceptions about adverse events, and the arguments and explanations against those misconceptions are noted in parentheses:

- "Bad apples" or incompetent health care providers are a common cause. (Although human error is commonly an initiating event, the faulty process of delivering care invariably permits or compounds the harm, and is the focus of improvement.

- High risk procedures or medical specialties are responsible for most *avoidable* adverse events. (Although some mistakes, such as in surgery, are harder to conceal, errors occur in all levels of care. Even though complex procedures entail more risk, adverse outcomes are not usually due to error, but to the severity of the condition being treated.). However, USP has reported that medication errors during the course of a surgical procedure are three times more likely to cause harm to a patient than those occurring in other types of hospital care.

- If a patient experiences an adverse event during the process of care, an error has occurred. (Most medical care entails some level of risk, and there can be complications or side effects, even unforeseen ones, from the underlying condition or from the treatment itself.)

Computerized Provider Order Entry

Computerized physician order entry (CPOE), sometimes referred to as computerized provider order entry or computerized provider order management (CPOM), is a process of electronic entry of medical practitioner instructions for the treatment of patients (particularly hospitalized patients) under his or her care.

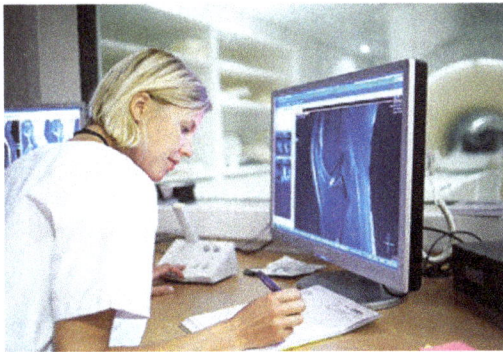

The entered orders are communicated over a computer network to the medical staff or to the departments (pharmacy, laboratory, or radiology) responsible for fulfilling the order. CPOE reduces the time it takes to distribute and complete orders, while increasing efficiency by reducing transcription errors including preventing duplicate order entry, while simplifying inventory management and billing.

CPOE is a form of patient management software.

Required Data

In a graphical representation of an order sequence, specific data should be presented to CPOE system staff in cleartext, including:

- Identity of the patient
- Role of required member of staff
- Resources, materials and medication applied
- Procedures to be performed
- Operational sequence to be obeyed
- Feedback to be noted
- Case specific documentation to build.

Some textual data can be reduced to simple graphics.

CPOE Related Terminology

CPOE systems use terminology familiar to medical and nursing staff, but there are different terms used to classify and concatenate orders. The following items are examples of additional terminology that a CPOE system programmer might need to know:

Filler

The application responding to, *i.e.*, performing, a request for services (orders) or producing an observation. The filler can also originate requests for services (new orders), add additional services to existing orders, replace existing orders, put an order on hold, discontinue an order, release a held order, or cancel existing orders.

Order

A request for a service from one application to a second application. In some cases an application is allowed to place orders with itself.

Order Detail Segment

One of several segments that can carry order information. Future ancillary specific segments may be defined in subsequent releases of the Standard if they become necessary.

Placer

The application or individual originating a request for services (order).

Placer Order Group

A list of associated orders coming from a single location regarding a single patient.

Order Set

A grouping of orders used to standardize and expedite the ordering process for a common clinical scenario. (Typically, these orders are started, modified, and stopped by a licensed physician.)

Protocol

A grouping of orders used to standardize and automate a clinical process on behalf of a physician. (Typically, these orders are started, modified, and stopped by a nurse, pharmacist, or other licensed health professional.)

Features of CPOE Systems

Features of the ideal computerized physician order entry system (CPOE) include:

- Ordering

  Physician orders are standardized across the organization, yet may be individualized for each doctor or specialty by using order sets. Orders are communicated to all departments and involved caregivers, improving response time and avoiding scheduling problems and conflict with existing orders.

- Patient-Centered Decision Support

  The ordering process includes a display of the patient's medical history and current results and evidence-based clinical guidelines to support treatment decisions. Often uses medical logic module and/or Arden syntax to facilitate fully integrated Clinical Decision Support Systems (CDSS).

- Patient Safety Features

  The CPOE system allows real-time patient identification, drug dose recommendations; adverse drug reaction reviews, and checks on allergies and test or treatment conflicts. Physicians and nurses can review orders immediately for confirmation.

- Intuitive Human Interface

  The order entry workflow corresponds to familiar "paper-based" ordering to allow efficient use by new or infrequent users.

- Regulatory Compliance and Security

  Access is secure, and a permanent record is created, with electronic signature.

- Portability

  The system accepts and manages orders for all departments at the point-of-care, from any location in the health system (physician's office, hospital or home) through a variety of devices, including wireless PCs and tablet computers.

- Management

  The system delivers statistical reports online so that managers can analyze patient census and make changes in staffing, replace inventory and audit utilization and productivity throughout the organization. Data is collected for training, planning, and root cause analysis for patient safety events.

- Billing

  Documentation is improved by linking diagnoses (ICD-9-CM or ICD-10-CM codes) to orders at the time of order entry to support appropriate charges.

Patient Safety Benefits

In the past, physicians have traditionally hand-written or verbally communicated orders for patient care, which are then transcribed by various individuals (such as unit clerks, nurses, and ancillary staff) before being carried out. Handwritten reports or notes, manual order entry, non-standard abbreviations and poor legibility lead to errors and injuries to patients, . A follow up IOM report in 2001 advised use of electronic medication ordering, with computer- and internet-based information systems to support clinical decisions. Prescribing errors are the largest identified source of preventable hospital medical error. A 2006 report by the Institute of Medicine estimated that a hospitalized patient is exposed to a medication error each day of his or her stay. While further studies have estimated that CPOE implementation at all nonrural hospitals in the United States could prevent over 500,000 serious medication errors each year. Studies of computerized physician order entry (CPOE) has yielded evidence that suggests the medication error rate can be reduced by 80%, and errors that have potential for serious harm or death for patients can be reduced by 55%, and other studies have also suggested benefits. Further, in 2005, CMS and CDC released a report that showed only 41 percent of prophylactic antibacterial were correctly stopped within 24 hours of completed surgery. The researchers conducted an analysis over an eight-month period, implementing a CPOE system designed to stop the administration of prophylactic antibacterials. Results showed CPOE significantly improved timely discontinuation of antibacterials from 38.8 percent of surgeries to 55.7 percent in the intervention hospital. CPOE/e-Prescribing systems can provide automatic dosing alerts (for example, letting the user know that the dose is too high and thus dangerous) and interaction checking (for example, telling the user that 2 medicines ordered taken together can cause health problems). In this way, specialists in pharmacy informatics work with the medical and nursing staffs at hospitals to improve the safety and effectiveness of medication use by utilizing CPOE systems.

Advantages

Generally, CPOE is advantageous, as it leaves the trails of just better formatting retrospective information, as with traditional hospital information systems designs. The key advantage of providing information from the physician in charge of treatment for a single patient to the different roles involved in processing he treatise itself is widely innovative. This makes CPOE the primary tool for information transfer to the performing staff and lesser the tool for collecting action items for the accounting staff. However, the needs of proper accounting get served automatically upon feedback on completion of orders.

CPOE is generally not suitable without reasonable training and tutoring respectively. As with other technical means, the system based communicating of information may be inaccessible or inoperable due to failures. That is not different to making use of an ordinary telephone or with conventional hospital information systems. Beyond, the information conveyed may be faulty or erratic. A concatenated validating of orders must be well organized. Errors lead to liability cases as with all professional treatment of patients.

Prescriber and staff inexperience may cause slower entry of orders at first, use more staff time, and is slower than person-to-person communication in an emergency situation. Physician to nurse communication can worsen if each group works alone at their workstations.

But, in general, the options to reuse order sets anew with new patients lays the basic for substantial enhancement of the processing of services to the patients in the complex distribution of work amongst the roles involved. The basic concepts are defined with the clinical pathway approach. However, success does not occur by itself. The preparatory work has to be budgeted from the very beginning and has to be maintained all the time. Patterns of proper management from other service industry and from production industry may apply. However, the medical methodologies and nursing procedures do not get affected by the management approaches.

Risks

CPOE presents several possible dangers by introducing new types of errors. Automation causes a false sense of security, a misconception that when technology suggests a course of action, errors are avoided. These factors contributed to an *increased* mortality rate in the Children's Hospital of Pittsburgh's Pediatric ICU when a CPOE systems was introduced. In other settings, shortcut or default selections can override non-standard medication regimens for elderly or underweight patients, resulting in toxic doses.

Frequent alerts and warnings can interrupt work flow, causing these messages to be ignored or overridden due to alert fatigue. CPOE and automated drug dispensing was identified as a cause of error by 84% of over 500 health care facilities participating in a surveillance system by the United States Pharmacopoeia. Introducing CPOE to a complex medical environment requires ongoing changes in design to cope with unique patients and care settings, close supervision of overrides caused by automatic systems, and training, testing and re-training all users.

Implementation

CPOE systems can take years to install and configure. Despite ample evidence of the potential to reduce medication errors, adoption of this technology by doctors and hospitals in the United States has been slowed by resistance to changes in physician's practice patterns, costs and training time involved, and concern with interoperability and compliance with future national standards. According to a study by RAND Health, the US healthcare system could save more than 81 billion dollars annually, reduce adverse medical events and improve the quality of care if it were to widely adopt CPOE and other health information technology. As more hospitals become aware of the financial benefits of CPOE, and more physicians with a familiarity with computers enter practice, increased use of CPOE is predicted. Several high-profile failures of CPOE implementation have occurred, so a major effort must be focused on change management, including restructuring workflows, dealing with physicians' resistance to change, and creating a collaborative environment.

An early success with CPOE by the United States Department of Veterans Affairs (VA) is the Veterans Health Information Systems and Technology Architecture or VistA. A graphical user interface known as the Computerized Patient Record System (CPRS) allows health care providers to review and update a patient's record at any computer in the VA's over 1,000 healthcare facilities. CPRS includes the ability to place orders by CPOE, including medications, special procedures, x-rays, patient care nursing orders, diets and laboratory tests.

The world's first successful implementation of a CPOE system was at El Camino Hospital in Mountain View, California in the early 1970s. The Medical Information System (MIS) was originally developed by a software and hardware team at Lockheed in Sunnyvale, California, which became the TMIS group at Technicon Instruments Corporation. The MIS system used a light pen to allow physicians and nurses to quickly point and click items to be ordered.

As of 2005, one of the largest projects for a national EHR is by the National Health Service (NHS) in the United Kingdom. The goal of the NHS is to have 60,000,000 patients with a centralized electronic health record by 2010. The plan involves a gradual roll-out commencing May 2006, providing general practices in England access to the National Programme for IT (NPfIT). The NHS component, known as the "Connecting for Health

Programme", includes office-based CPOE for medication prescribing and test ordering and retrieval, although some concerns have been raised about patient safety features.

In 2008, the Massachusetts Technology Collaborative and the New England Health-care Institute (NEHI) published research showing that 1 in 10 patients admitted to a Massachusetts community hospital suffered a preventable medication error. The study argued that Massachusetts hospitals could prevent 55,000 adverse drug events per year and save $170 million annually if they fully implemented CPOE. The findings prompted the Commonwealth of Massachusetts to enact legislation requiring all hospitals to implement CPOE by 2012 as a condition of licensure.

In addition, the study also concludes that it would cost approximately $2.1 million to implement a CPOE system, and a cost of $435,000 to maintain it in the state of Massachusetts while it saves annually about $2.7 million per hospital. The hospitals will still see payback within 26 months through reducing hospitalizations generated by error. Despite the advantages and cost savings, the CPOE is still not well adapted by many hospitals in the US.

The Leapfrog's 2008 Survey showed that most hospitals are still not complying with having a fully implemented, effective CPOE system. The CPOE requirement became more challenging to meet in 2008 because the Leapfrog introduced a new requirement: Hospitals must test their CPOE systems with Leapfrog's CPOE Evaluation Tool. So the number of hospitals in the survey considered to be fully meeting the standard dropped to 7% in 2008 from 11% the previous year. Though the adoption rate seems very low in 2008, it is still an improvement from 2002 when only 2% of hospitals met this Leapfrog standard.

Evidence-based Medicine

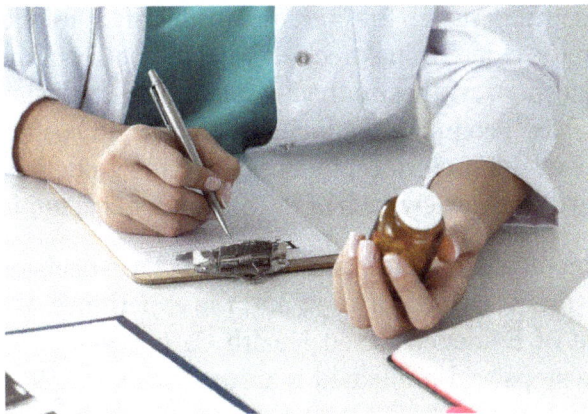

Evidence based medicine (EBM) is the conscientious, explicit, judicious and reasonable use of modern, best evidence in making decisions about the care of individual patients. EBM integrates clinical experience and patient values with the best available research information. It is a movement which aims to increase the use of high quality clinical research in clinical decision making.

Skills that all Practicing EBM Clinicians really Need

While EBM is a large step forward, these skills are necessary but not sufficient for the practice of contemporary medicine. All clinicians should:

- Find the best evidence for every day practice (Information mastery).

- Assess relevance before rigor. Is the evidence patient oriented?

- Evaluate information about therapies, diagnostic tests, and clinicaldecision rules. Is it true?

- Understand basic statistics.

- Have at fingertips "just in time" information at the point of care using web based and/or handheld computer based information and tools for clinical decision making.

- Evaluate expert-based information, including colleagues, CME, presentations, reviews and guidelines.

- Critically evaluate information from pharmaceutical representatives.

Methods

Steps

The steps for designing explicit, evidence-based guidelines were described in the late 1980s: Formulate the question (population, intervention, comparison intervention, outcomes, time horizon, setting); search the literature to identify studies that inform the question; interpret each study to determine precisely what it says about the question; if several studies address the question, synthesize their results (meta-analysis); summarize the evidence in "evidence tables"; compare the benefits, harms and costs in a "balance sheet"; draw a conclusion about the preferred practice; write the guideline; write the rationale for the guideline; have others review each of the previous steps; implement the guideline.

For the purposes of medical education and individual-level decision making, five steps of EBM in practice were described in 1992 and the experience of delegates attending the 2003 Conference of Evidence-Based Health Care Teachers and Developers was summarized into five steps and published in 2005. This five step process can broadly be categorized as:

1. Translation of uncertainty to an answerable question and includes critical questioning, study design and levels of evidence.

2. Systematic retrieval of the best evidence available.

3. Critical appraisal of evidence for internal validity that can be broken down into aspects regarding:

    ◦   Systematic errors as a result of selection bias, information bias and confounding.

    ◦   Quantitative aspects of diagnosis and treatment.

    ◦   The effect size and aspects regarding its precision.

    ◦   Clinical importance of results.

    ◦   External validity or generalizability.

4. Application of results in practice.

5. Evaluation of performance.

Evidence Reviews

Systematic reviews of published research studies is a major part of the evaluation of particular treatments. The Cochrane Collaboration is one of the best-known programs that conducts systematic reviews. Like other collections of systematic reviews, it requires authors to provide a detailed and repeatable plan of their literature search and evaluations of the evidence. Once all the best evidence is assessed, treatment is categorized as:

1. Likely to be beneficial,

2. Likely to be harmful, or

3. Evidence did not support either benefit or harm.

A 2007 analysis of 1,016 systematic reviews from all 50 Cochrane Collaboration Review Groups found that 44% of the reviews concluded that the intervention was likely to be beneficial, 7% concluded that the intervention was likely to be harmful, and 49% concluded that evidence did not support either benefit or harm. 96% recommended further research. A 2001 review of 160 Cochrane systematic reviews (excluding complementary treatments) in the 1998 database revealed that, according to two readers, 41% concluded positive or possibly positive effect, 20% concluded evidence of no effect, 8% concluded net harmful effects, and 21% of the reviews concluded insufficient evidence. A review of 145 alternative medicine Cochrane reviews using the 2004 database revealed that 38.4% concluded positive effect or possibly positive (12.4%) effect, 4.8% concluded no effect, 0.7% concluded harmful effect, and 56.6% concluded insufficient evidence. In 2017, a study assessed the role of systematic reviews produced by

Cochrane Collaboration to inform US private payers' policies making; it showed that though medical policy documents of major US private were informed by Cochrane systematic review; there was still scope to encourage the further usage.

Assessing the Quality of Evidence

Evidence quality can be assessed based on the source type (from meta-analyses and systematic reviews of triple-blind randomized clinical trials with concealment of allocation and no attrition at the top end, down to conventional wisdom at the bottom), as well as other factors including statistical validity, clinical relevance, currency, and peer-review acceptance. Evidence-based medicine categorizes different types of clinical evidence and rates or grades them according to the strength of their freedom from the various biases that beset medical research. For example, the strongest evidence for therapeutic interventions is provided by systematic review of randomized, triple-blind, placebo-controlled trials with allocation concealment and complete follow-up involving a homogeneous patient population and medical condition. In contrast, patient testimonials, case reports, and even expert opinion (however, some critics have argued that expert opinion "does not belong in the rankings of the quality of empirical evidence because it does not represent a form of empirical evidence" and continue that "expert opinion would seem to be a separate, complex type of knowledge that would not fit into hierarchies otherwise limited to empirical evidence alone"). have little value as proof because of the placebo effect, the biases inherent in observation and reporting of cases, difficulties in ascertaining who is an expert and more.

Several organizations have developed grading systems for assessing the quality of evidence. For example, in 1989 the U.S. Preventive Services Task Force (USPSTF) put forth the following:

- Level I: Evidence obtained from at least one properly designed randomized controlled trial.

- Level II-1: Evidence obtained from well-designed controlled trials without randomization.

- Level II-2: Evidence obtained from well-designed cohort studies or case-control studies, preferably from more than one center or research group.

- Level II-3: Evidence obtained from multiple time series designs with or without the intervention. Dramatic results in uncontrolled trials might also be regarded as this type of evidence.

- Level III: Opinions of respected authorities, based on clinical experience, descriptive studies, or reports of expert committees.

Another example is the Oxford (UK) CEBM Levels of Evidence. First released in September 2000, the Oxford CEBM Levels of Evidence provides 'levels' of evidence for claims about prognosis, diagnosis, treatment benefits, treatment harms, and screening, which most grading schemes do not address. The original CEBM Levels was Evidence-Based On Call to make the process of finding evidence feasible and its results explicit. In 2011, an international team redesigned the Oxford CEBM Levels to make it more understandable and to take into account recent developments in evidence ranking schemes. The Oxford CEBM Levels of Evidence have been used by patients, clinicians and also to develop clinical guidelines including recommendations for the optimal use of phototherapy and topical therapy in psoriasis and guidelines for the use of the BCLC staging system for diagnosing and monitoring hepatocellular carcinoma in Canada.

In 2000, a system was developed by the GRADE (short for Grading of Recommendations Assessment, Development and Evaluation) working group and takes into account more dimensions than just the quality of medical research. It requires users of GRADE who are performing an assessment of the quality of evidence, usually as part of a systematic review, to consider the impact of different factors on their confidence in the results. Authors of GRADE tables grade the quality of evidence into four levels, on the basis of their confidence in the observed effect (a numerical value) being close to what the true effect is. The confidence value is based on judgements assigned in five different domains in a structured manner. The GRADE working group defines 'quality of evidence' and 'strength of recommendations' based on the quality as two different concepts which are commonly confused with each other.

Systematic reviews may include randomized controlled trials that have low risk of bias, or, observational studies that have high risk of bias. In the case of randomized controlled trials, the quality of evidence is high, but can be downgraded in five different domains.

- Risk of bias: is a judgement made on the basis of the chance that bias in included studies has influenced the estimate of effect.

- Imprecision: is a judgement made on the basis of the chance that the observed estimate of effect could change completely.

- Indirectness: is a judgement made on the basis of the differences in characteristics of how the study was conducted and how the results are actually going to be applied.

- Inconsistency: is a judgement made on the basis of the variability of results across the included studies.

- Publication bias: is a judgement made on the basis of the question whether all the research evidence has been taken to account.

In the case of observational studies per GRADE, the quality of evidence starts of lower and may be upgraded in three domains in addition to being subject to downgrading.

- Large effect: This is when methodologically strong studies show that the observed effect is so large that the probability of it changing completely is less likely.

- Plausible confounding would change the effect: This is when despite the presence of a possible confounding factor which is expected to reduce the observed effect, the effect estimate still shows significant effect.

- Dose response gradient: This is when the intervention used becomes more effective with increasing dose. This suggests that a further increase will likely bring about more effect.

Meaning of the levels of quality of evidence as per GRADE:

- High Quality Evidence: The authors are very confident that the estimate that is presented lies very close to the true value. One could interpret it as "there is very low probability of further research completely changing the presented conclusions."

- Moderate Quality Evidence: The authors are confident that the presented estimate lies close to the true value, but it is also possible that it may be substantially different. One could also interpret it as: further research may completely change the conclusions.

- Low Quality Evidence: The authors are not confident in the effect estimate and the true value may be substantially different. One could interpret it as "further research is likely to change the presented conclusions completely."

- Very low quality Evidence: The authors do not have any confidence in the estimate and it is likely that the true value is substantially different from it. One could interpret it as "new research will most probably change the presented conclusions completely."

Categories of Recommendations

In guidelines and other publications, recommendation for a clinical service is classified by the balance of risk versus benefit and the level of evidence on which this information is based. The U.S. Preventive Services Task Force uses:

- Level A: Good scientific evidence suggests that the benefits of the clinical service substantially outweigh the potential risks. Clinicians should discuss the service with eligible patients.

- Level B: At least fair scientific evidence suggests that the benefits of the clinical service outweigh the potential risks. Clinicians should discuss the service with eligible patients.

- Level C: At least fair scientific evidence suggests that there are benefits provided by the clinical service, but the balance between benefits and risks are too close for making general recommendations. Clinicians need not offer it unless there are individual considerations.

- Level D: At least fair scientific evidence suggests that the risks of the clinical service outweigh potential benefits. Clinicians should not routinely offer the service to asymptomatic patients.

- Level I: Scientific evidence is lacking, of poor quality, or conflicting, such that the risk versus benefit balance cannot be assessed. Clinicians should help patients understand the uncertainty surrounding the clinical service.

GRADE guideline panelists may make strong or weak recommendations on the basis of further criteria. Some of the important criteria are the balance between desirable and undesirable effects (not considering cost), the quality of the evidence, values and preferences and costs (resource utilization).

Despite the differences between systems, the purposes are the same: to guide users of clinical research information on which studies are likely to be most valid. However, the individual studies still require careful critical appraisal.

Statistical Measures

Evidence-based medicine attempts to express clinical benefits of tests and treatments using mathematical methods. Tools used by practitioners of evidence-based medicine include:

- Likelihood ratio :The pre-test odds of a particular diagnosis, multiplied by the likelihood ratio, determines the post-test odds. (Odds can be calculated from, and then converted to, the [more familiar] probability.) This reflects Bayes' theorem. The differences in likelihood ratio between clinical tests can be used to prioritize clinical tests according to their usefulness in a given clinical situation.

- AUC-ROC: The area under the receiver operating characteristic curve (AUC-ROC) reflects the relationship between sensitivity and specificity for a given test. High-quality tests will have an AUC-ROC approaching 1, and high-quality publications about clinical tests will provide information about the AUC-ROC. Cutoff values for positive and negative tests can influence specificity and sensitivity, but they do not affect AUC-ROC.

- Number needed to treat (NNT)/Number needed to harm (NNH): Number needed to treat or number needed to harm are ways of expressing the effectiveness and safety, respectively, of interventions in a way that is clinically meaningful. NNT is the number of people who need to be treated in order to achieve the desired outcome (e.g. survival from cancer) in one patient. For example, if a treatment increases the chance of survival by 5%, then 20 people need to be treated in order to have 1 additional patient survive due to the treatment. The concept can also be applied to diagnostic tests. For example, if 1339 women age 50–59 have to be invited for breast cancer screening over a ten-year period in order to prevent one woman from dying of breast cancer, then the NNT for being invited to breast cancer screening is 1339.

Quality of Clinical Trials

Evidence-based medicine attempts to objectively evaluate the quality of clinical research by critically assessing techniques reported by researchers in their publications.

- Trial design considerations. High-quality studies have clearly defined eligibility criteria and have minimal missing data.

- Generalizability considerations. Studies may only be applicable to narrowly defined patient populations and may not be generalizable to other clinical contexts.

- Follow-up. Sufficient time for defined outcomes to occur can influence the prospective study outcomes and the statistical power of a study to detect differences between a treatment and control arm.

- Power. A mathematical calculation can determine if the number of patients is sufficient to detect a difference between treatment arms. A negative study may reflect a lack of benefit, or simply a lack of sufficient quantities of patients to detect a difference.

Electronic Health Record

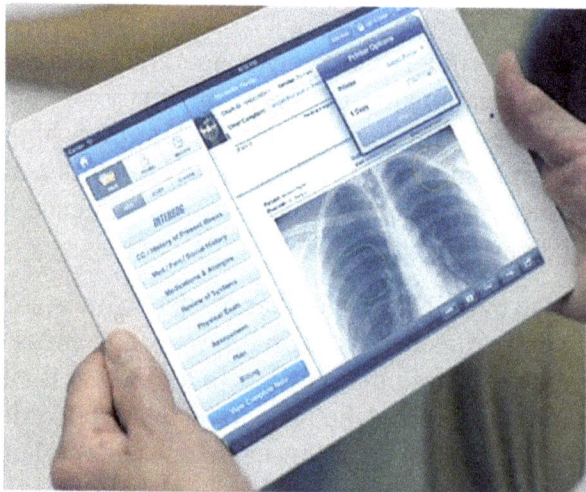

An electronic health record (EHR) is an automated, paperless and online medical record for which patient medical data is entered by eligible providers (EP), such as nurses and physicians. An EHR contains valuable and pertinent automated medical information, including:

- Patient vitals

- Prescriptions

- Medical histories

- Diagnoses

- Surgical notes

- Discharge summaries.

While EHRs are meant to be shared by EPs for enhanced patient treatment and less human medical error, as well as cost containment, many EHR concerns and complexities arise when considering privacy issues, especially regarding sensitive health data, such as behavioral health information. Electronic health records are also known as electronic medical records (EMR).

Electronic health records may be viewed by other patient care EPs, as well as patients. Although EHRs are designed to further interoperability or health information exchanges (HIE), IT personnel must work to tailor databases to prevent the automatic release of sensitive data for the preservation of doctor-patient relationships, as well as secure data to prevent release to marketing firms and malicious types of unauthorized users. Privacy advocates believe EHR vendors do not provide proper database security. To combat this serious issue, privacy protection laws are continuously gaining legislative support, as existing regulations do not entirely take into account protected health information (PHI).

EHR implementation is required by law under the American Recovery and Reinvestment Act (ARRA) of 2009, also known as the Stimulus Act, by the year 2015, for all U.S. health care organizations claiming Medicare/Medicaid reimbursement and incentive payments. Many expect this deadline to be extended due to the difficulty of nationwide implementation. Those that find EHR implementation most arduous are small private practices without ample IT resources and rural-based health facilities. EHR implementation began long before legislative requirements were established for teaching hospitals, large enterprises and other health care organizations that typically have a plethora of IT professionals.

References

- Institute of Medicine (2000). To Err Is Human: Building a Safer Health System. Washington, DC: The National Academies Press. doi:10.17226/9728. ISBN 978-0-309-26174-6

- What-exactly-is-patient-advocacy: rncentral.com, Retrieved 12 July 2018

- Leape LL (1994). "Error in medicine". JAMA. 272 (23): 1851–7. doi:10.1001/jama.272.23.1851. PMID 7503827.

- Medical-errors-causes-solutions: scribeamerica.com, Retrieved 28 May 2018

- Friedman, Richard A.; D, M (2003). "CASES; Do Spelling and Penmanship Count? In Medicine, You Bet". The New York Times. Retrieved 2018-08-29.

- Electronic-health-record-her-15337: techopedia.com, Retrieved 11 April 2018

- "Incorporating Patient-Safe Design into the Guidelines". The American Institute of Architects Academy Journal. The American Institute of Architects. 2005-10-19.

Permissions

All chapters in this book are published with permission under the Creative Commons Attribution Share Alike License or equivalent. Every chapter published in this book has been scrutinized by our experts. Their significance has been extensively debated. The topics covered herein carry significant information for a comprehensive understanding. They may even be implemented as practical applications or may be referred to as a beginning point for further studies.

We would like to thank the editorial team for lending their expertise to make the book truly unique. They have played a crucial role in the development of this book. Without their invaluable contributions this book wouldn't have been possible. They have made vital efforts to compile up to date information on the varied aspects of this subject to make this book a valuable addition to the collection of many professionals and students.

This book was conceptualized with the vision of imparting up-to-date and integrated information in this field. To ensure the same, a matchless editorial board was set up. Every individual on the board went through rigorous rounds of assessment to prove their worth. After which they invested a large part of their time researching and compiling the most relevant data for our readers.

The editorial board has been involved in producing this book since its inception. They have spent rigorous hours researching and exploring the diverse topics which have resulted in the successful publishing of this book. They have passed on their knowledge of decades through this book. To expedite this challenging task, the publisher supported the team at every step. A small team of assistant editors was also appointed to further simplify the editing procedure and attain best results for the readers.

Apart from the editorial board, the designing team has also invested a significant amount of their time in understanding the subject and creating the most relevant covers. They scrutinized every image to scout for the most suitable representation of the subject and create an appropriate cover for the book.

The publishing team has been an ardent support to the editorial, designing and production team. Their endless efforts to recruit the best for this project, has resulted in the accomplishment of this book. They are a veteran in the field of academics and their pool of knowledge is as vast as their experience in printing. Their expertise and guidance has proved useful at every step. Their uncompromising quality standards have made this book an exceptional effort. Their encouragement from time to time has been an inspiration for everyone.

The publisher and the editorial board hope that this book will prove to be a valuable piece of knowledge for students, practitioners and scholars across the globe.

Index